M000041288

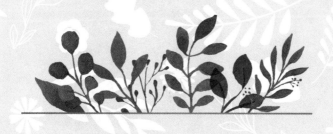

Mindful Mama

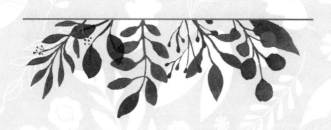

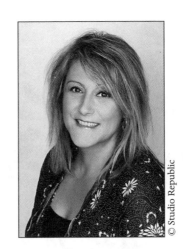

About the Author

Ileana Abrev is the bestselling author of three New Age books. With knowledge passed down to her by her father, an esteemed spiritual medium, Ileana guides her clients on a daily basis to solve problems while assisting them with manifesting positive outcomes. She lives in Queensland, Australia.

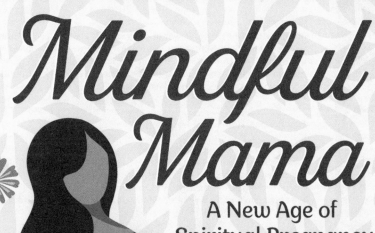

Mindful Mama

A New Age of
Spiritual Pregnancy

Ileana Abrev

Llewellyn Publications
Woodbury, Minnesota

FIRST EDITION
First Printing, 2020

Book design by Donna Burch-Brown
Cover design by Shira Atakpu
Editing by Rhiannon Nelson
Interior art design by Llewellyn Art Department
Llewellyn Publications is a registered trademark of Llewellyn Worldwide
    Ltd.

Library of Congress Cataloging-in-Publication Data
Names: Abrev, Ileana, author.
Title: Mindful mama : a new age of spiritual pregnancy / Ileana Abrev.
Description: Woodbury, Minnesota : Llewellyn Worldwide, [2020]
Identifiers: LCCN 2020016954 (print) | LCCN 2020016955 (ebook) | ISBN
    9780738762463 (paperback) | ISBN 9780738762531 (ebook)
Subjects: LCSH: Pregnancy—Popular works.
Classification: LCC RG525 .A25 2020 (print) | LCC RG525 (ebook) | DDC
    618.2—dc23
LC record available at https://lccn.loc.gov/2020016954
LC ebook record available at https://lccn.loc.gov/2020016955

Llewellyn Publications
A Division of Llewellyn Worldwide Ltd.
2143 Wooddale Drive
Woodbury, MN 55125-2989
www.llewellyn.com
Printed in the United States of America

Other Books by Ileana Abrev

The Little Brown Book of White Spells
A Cart Full of Magic

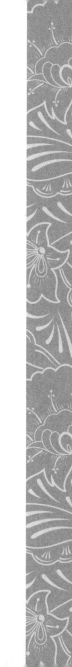

Disclaimer

This book is not intended to provide medical advice or to take the place of medical advice and treatment from your healthcare professionals. Readers are advised to consult their qualified healthcare professionals regarding their care. Neither the publisher nor the author takes any responsibility for any possible consequences from any treatment, action, or application of medicine, supplement, herb, technique, or preparation to any person reading or following the information in this book.

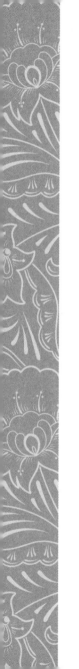

Dedication

To the mother-to-be, here is to a mindful pregnancy.
To my kids, Beverly and Ben, I love you dearly.

Contents

Part Two—First Trimester

Part Three—Second Trimester

Part Four—Third Trimester

Part Five—Birthing and Beyond

Introduction

This book is about being spiritually in tune with the essence of your unborn child, from conception to the end of your pregnancy, while creating a positive womb experience that will carry your child into adulthood.

While there are many books full of medical advice for pregnant women, *Mindful Mama* is not one of them, and it should never be a substitute for prenatal care with your chosen medical provider. This book is a spiritual medium to bring you peace while pregnant, keep you calm in stressful situations, keep you grounded and focused, and most important, connect you with your baby.

Using *Mindful Mama* to elevate your mood and lighten your load can make this wonderful journey more fulfilling. When used in conjunction with other books that concentrate on practical advice discussing diet, nutrition, and prenatal care, it will not only be more fulfilling for your physical and mental health, but also the well-being of your baby.

We know a lot and at the same time we know little of what actually happens from conception to the end of the gestation period. At the same time, we are often taken by surprise by some of the things that happen during pregnancy. Medical issues can crop up during your pregnancy that need attention and follow-up with your medical provider. While you encounter all the things that happen during pregnancy, *Mindful Mama* will keep you spiritually aware and positive.

While pregnant, you'll want to treasure and cherish every second of this rite of passage, not only for yourself, but also for the little human growing within you. You'll want to create a womb experience that is filled with love and free of the stress we often encounter each day.

You want to give your pregnancy the best care you can possibly give it. You may even feel a little scared. How can you not be? Your mind may flow from one thing to another, untamed at not knowing how good of a mother you will be. Understanding the responsibility that comes with the mother role and accepting that it is yours until the end of your time on this plane of existence can be overwhelming, exciting, mortifying, and even moving.

The connection you forge with your unborn child is precious. You want to retain every minute of this connection as your child grows and prospers within your womb. If this is not your first pregnancy, you know how quickly the weeks pass. Before you know it, you're in the delivery room having your baby.

Before this happens and you are whisked away to the delivery room, you want to remember every single aspect of your pregnancy. You want to remember morning sickness. I know, who wants to remember that? But it is memorable in a not-so-memorable way. And it's likely one of the first things you will associate with your first trimester after the joy of finding out you're pregnant.

You want to feel every kick and hold on to every movement to remember it. You want to give your baby the ability to make good choices in the future, to be their own person, and to have a dependable outlook on a life that is full of possibilities and self-worth. Not only as your baby grows from a baby to a child to an adult, but also throughout your pregnancy.

Mindful Mama is more than a pregnancy book; it is a spiritual journey for both you and your developing baby. This journey can help you create a life that grows into a strong adult with a positive outlook on life and who is not afraid to go for what he or she wants while navigating life's challenges.

This book will help you develop your own Goddess energy. And remember that pregnancy is not a disease; it doesn't stop you from doing all the things you were already enjoying. Just keep in mind there are restrictions that you should always adhere to, outlined by your medical practitioner. When you follow these instructions, the journey can be very rewarding.

If you want a better relationship with your child than the one you had with your parents, this book is worth reading. If you want your baby to feel comfortable and happy to have you and your partner as parents and to be a part of your family, then you are on the right track.

About the Book

This book helps you stay focused on what can go right throughout the growth and development of your baby growing within you. This book covers every stage of your pregnancy, and helps you navigate the challenges within each trimester, including work and family issues, self-image, choosing names, gender disappointment, sharing womb space, stress, and even choosing the color for your baby's room.

Addressing each stage of your pregnancy helps you cope, understand, and maintain the physical and emotional balance that can have you feeling blissful one minute and filled with insecurities the next. Be assured that you will find the connection you seek to actively interact with your baby to keep you both enlightened throughout the journey.

Mindful Mama is sectioned into five parts, which are easy to follow and essential to this amazing and wondrous journey. In part 1, Alliance of Energies, I introduce the Mindful Tools like crystals, essential oils, flowers, candles, and soothing baths. Then we dive into the Mindful Allies such as affirmations, meditation, and positive visualization. By actively using these Mindful Tools and Allies together, you will take your pregnancy to a higher level of consciousness for you and your child.

By using these Mindful Allies and Tools and saying something as simple as *"You will navigate life's problems with ease and comfort"* during your baby's growth cycle, you are setting your child to work through problems in the future with ease and comfort.

You will use these Mindful Tools and Allies during all the trimesters. Part 2 takes you from conception to the end of week 12 of the first trimester. Part 3 covers weeks 13 to 26 of the second trimester, and Part 4 discusses week 27 to week 40 of the third trimester.

Within each week in parts 2, 3, and 4, the baby's development is outlined. We will also cover what emotions you may be experiencing and how to enhance your baby's growth and spiritual development during that week. For example, the kidneys are part of the sacral chakra and are used for filtering within the body. By strengthening your child's kidneys during your pregnancy, you give your child a positive adulthood where they can filter anger, resentment, and even bitterness, which could be spiritual toxins in your child's future.

Each week I will show you how to use the Mindful Tools and Allies' energies—such as candles, baths, flowers, crystals, safe essential oils, meditations, affirmations, and visualizations—to create a positive outcome as each stage of your pregnancy is addressed and revealed. There will also be Mindful Hints and Mindful Moments throughout the book to help you cope with everyday pregnancy issues that you may encounter.

Part 5 covers the birth until you bring your baby home, plus other Mindful Hints and extras to look back on as a reference, such star signs, birthstones, and past-life memories.

Mindful Mama is your spiritual guide during this magical journey of creating life. Keep it by your bedside, the coffee table in your living room, or in your kitchen for easy access. Highlight areas you want to remember or address later in your pregnancy, or bookmark a positive affirmation you want to use as your pregnancy mantra throughout the journey.

You will find that *Mindful Mama* is an interactive, hands-on guide to participate in the growth and development of your baby, as well as the mother you are about to become.

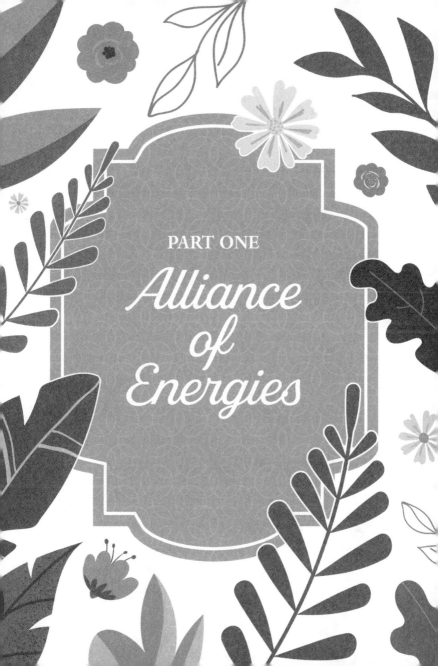

PART ONE

*Alliance
of
Energies*

Commitment

The journey of creating and nurturing life does not only encompass the nine months of your pregnancy. It also entails you and your partner care for another little human being that will carry both of your DNA.

Having a child is a twenty-four-hour job, seven days a week. This is a job you don't get paid for; you do it out of love because there is no other way you would ever do it. You need the trust and support of the person that is going to be there for you and your child in the future, because without your partner's commitment, it's harder to do it on your own. And if difficult times arise, seek people within your support group to get you through.

There are also financial responsibilities and careers to consider, which only scratches the surface of the decisions you will encounter as parent. Families that require dual incomes keep growing due to the economy and our own personal needs, lifestyle, and, of course, keeping the roof over our heads.

Often careers or salaries determine if one parent can stay home with the baby. If neither parent can, the child will be placed in day care or with a family member or grandparent who can pick up the slack. Unfortunately, the maternal essence must work in unison with your financial responsibilities. This brings challenges that can start a war with the emotional part of the decision to have a baby. There is also the commitment you and your partner make to the pregnancy and the thereafter.

It's easy to bring a child into the world, but the hard work comes soon after the birth. If you or your partner can't agree on who will do the dishes before the baby is born, or if one partner never contributes, this will only get worse after the baby is born. Resentful feelings may start to surface and grow. Decision-making will get harder and harder when you start to parent. You want intimacy to mature and flourish with each decision you make, not to die or wilt because you and your partner can't agree.

When a decision is made, be happy about it. If it's decided you and your partner will do all household chores together, honor it. Don't do it for a month then stop. If you do, it will only bring further quarrels and bickering. Tackle the decision-making now and become partners in all things.

Communication is the best tool a relationship has to survive. Read parenting books so you don't go in blind. You'll find out there are diapers to change, feedings at all hours, and, yes, bouts of inexplicable crying. Then there are expenses like a reliable car, medical bills, diapers, clothes, shoes, school, and perhaps university in the future. Having open communication while making all these decisions will alleviate many problems, assumptions, or confusion that may arise.

Once you are both sure that having a baby is what you want, decisions become joy, joy becomes planning, and an exciting future is written. Remember, nothing is written in stone and everything that happens molds your family's future, so be open to altering your plans if need be.

Embrace your decision. Make a list of all the things a growing family needs to keep it materially and emotionally stable. Follow the list and cross out entries when they've been accomplished. Even if it takes you months or years to complete the list, it's there to remind you of the commitment you've made. Try to honor it for as long as it takes, no matter how many times you need to adjust things to complete your intention.

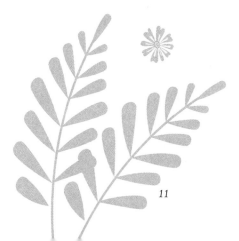

Mindful Tools and Allies

Mindful Tools are aids to our spiritual and physical needs and include things like crπystals, herbs,
essential oils, colors, flowers, and candles. Mindful
Allies are positive affirmations, meditation, spiritual-
ism, wisdom, and believing in oneself. We can tap into
any of the Mindful Allies whenever we seek spiritual
aid to manifest our deepest desires or lessen our stress.
We can utilize them to receive anything else we need
or want or use them to achieve our goals or get rid of
unwanted things in our life.

Mindful Tools are great conductors of energy.
They've been around as far back as when we started wor-
shipping the earth for our livelihood. They connect us
with universal forces as nothing else can. They belong
to the earth, fire, water, and air elements. They take
our needs where we want them to go by tapping into
our spiritual journey of consciousness, connecting our
desires, fears, and heartaches to find peace and comfort
within ourselves.

Without even knowing, we use these Mindful Tools,
some on a daily basis. There is always an odd candle
here and there throughout your house, the crystal you
carry or the one you have as an ornament. You might

have an essential oil hidden somewhere in a drawer or cabinet, perhaps lavender or a similar scent.

Using Mindful Allies while pregnant will help you stay grounded, remain positive, and above all unite you with your growing bundle. It will help you make that connection only a mother and her child will ever know. You can achieve this by using positive affirmations—meditations to enhance and enlighten your pregnancy to be a spiritually rewarding and fulfilling experience, a journey of everlasting love that is fulfilled with a lifetime of joy. By lighting a candle or using a crystal to stay positive and grounded, you will find a new sense of belief and strength to carry you through the journey you have embarked on. This makes one of the many connections you will have with your child throughout their life, even when they have families of their own.

When you bring the Mindful Tools and Allies together, you are not only connecting to your unborn child and creating an important emotional relationship that establishes peace and calm within the womb; you're also creating your child's future. These energies, together with mindfulness, bring forth a child that will be sure of the future they wish to have, a future that is without insecurities or reservations. Your child will be spirited, self-aware, even intuitive, just by blending Mindful Tools and Mindful Allies to shape their emotional future. And guess what? You are the vessel to their future.

Bringing these energies and mindfulness into your world causes a shift, and a new understanding of what is important and what really matters starts to stir deep within you. You begin to realize that cultivating awareness can actually lessen negative feelings, stress, and anxiety.

You and you alone choose the emotions you want your baby to have while in the womb. You want your baby to feel wanted, to feel peace, to feel safe in the living space you have provided. You want your baby to know that your uterus is a lovely and stable place to be. You want your baby to be assured that you have a positive emotional and healthy pregnancy.

And remember that when it comes to healthy pregnancies, whatever you eat is absorbed by your body and filters through your bloodstream to the baby via the placenta. This is why pregnant women should eat a well-balanced diet and should become familiar with the foods that are considered unsafe to eat while pregnant. Most important, women should abstain from drinking alcohol for the entire forty weeks of pregnancy and longer if they choose to breastfeed. Women do this to give their baby a healthy womb experience. Why not give your pregnancy emotional stability too? The baby feeds not only from their mother's physical nutrients, but from her emotional ones as well.

While Mindful Tools use living energies, Mindful Allies are there to help you remember to breathe, to think, and to not let the things you can't change upset you. Light a candle for spiritual guidance, play music that warms your soul, look at crystals to cause a positive effect, display flowers to warm your soul. Give yourself a daily positive affirmation, use safe essential oils, drink a cup of tea, meditate, keep your chakras balanced, and give into a carefree pregnancy that you'll forever cherish.

Throughout each week of your pregnancy, I will introduce you to the Mindful Tools and Allies, how to use them, and the benefits they can offer to your pregnancy. At the start of each trimester, there will be a list of the things you will need for that trimester so you can find the items and have them ready, even the flowers so you know when to get them and if they're in season.

Once you start to use the Mindful Tools and Allies, you will notice the difference within you. When you do, so will your child, and you'll carry them in a bubble of peace, love, and positive radiating energies, which brings a positive child to this plane of existence.

Mindful Tools

Chakras

The chakras are the seven life centers that reside deep within our spiritual body. Each one has a name, a color, and a crystal they vibrate to. They start at the base of your spine and finish at the top of your head. They embody our emotions, our health, and our spiritual awareness.

The first chakra is known as the root chakra. Its color is red, and it's located at the base of the spine. Its function is one of survival, the primal instinct of being human. This chakra is the most important for your growing baby. The root chakra is all about feeling secure, feeling grounded, and feeling safe. If you feel safe, so will your baby.

The second chakra is the sacral chakra and is found just below the belly button. Its color is orange and its function focuses on relationships, self-worth, sexual expression, beauty, creativity, and empathy. This chakra is mindful to accept new experiences during your pregnancy, even if it's not your first one.

From the belly button, we jump to the third chakra, the solar plexus. The color for the solar plexus is yellow and you'll find it between the breastbone and the belly button. Its function is power, self-awareness, intuition, trust, and self-esteem. This chakra is particularly mindful to prepare you for birth, giving you and your baby courage and spiritual strength.

The fourth life center is the heart chakra. You can find this chakra in the middle of your chest. Its color is green, and it expresses love, understanding, and compassion. This chakra is all about love for your baby and connecting to your baby. This chakra encompasses forgiveness and the hope for a lifetime connection to your child.

The throat chakra is the fifth chakra, and its color is blue. You can locate it at the center of your throat. This is the communication center of humanity and how we express ourselves with those around us. This chakra lets us listen and speak or write our fears and joys. This chakra will aid you in communicating with your partner during your pregnancy on the things that worry or scare you as well as communicating with your baby in utero.

The third eye is the sixth chakra and is located in the middle of your forehead. The third eye chakra is a brilliant purple and is all about wisdom and intuition and clarity of the mind. This chakra involves seeing the future—not in a divinatory way, but more intuitively. Balancing this chakra will help you make the right decisions throughout your pregnancy.

The seventh and last chakra is the crown chakra. This is on the crown or top of your head. The color is violet, white, and some perceive it as pink. This chakra is all about the higher truth, oneness, and spiritual transformation. This is the chakra to focus on when meditating to ground your pregnancy blessedness and to get in touch with your spiritual beliefs.

The chakras represent our emotional state, health, and balance of life. They are the psychic energy of our mind, body, and spirit. Those with intuitive sight have described them as colorful spinning wheels that are forever turning around each individual's center as it connects the Divine with the physical to create balance within each of us.

During your pregnancy, your chakras connect to the baby's chakras like an electrical current flowing back and forth between you and your baby. They connect until both energies are in tune with each other, but still leave each one with its own individuality. In the third trimester, the baby's first little chakra is formed, the root chakra. After the root chakra forms, four more chakras develop and look like flowers ready to bloom. It's believed the last two surface after birth, which focus on clarity and connectedness to the universe.

Harmonizing your chakras during pregnancy can help keep you grounded and emotionally balanced. I will guide you through each week by using affirmations that strengthen a particular life center to stay grounded, remain calm, and most important, stay connected to your pregnancy and the baby.

The way you treat yourself is the way you treat your child throughout your pregnancy. You want to pass positive energy to your baby; insecurities are in the *no-go* zone. This is because the chakras are on an emotional overload and overactive. They are working excessively—adjusting to the electrical energy forming within your womb that is forever growing and changing.

This is nothing short of a miracle.

The way you conduct yourself through pregnancy is a mirror image of what your child may one day turn out to be. You want your child to own their energy centers and be in tune with the person they'll one day be. By balancing your chakras, you will be able to give them the best start a parent could ever give their child: a future that is enriched with hope and assurance, all because of a well-balanced emotional womb experience.

Crystals

The collective influences of crystals are varied, but in general, crystals are protective and healing talismans that can transform your life and the needs of your growing baby. Once you tap into a crystal's unique beauty and strength, the effect is transformational, and this transformation becomes an excellent tool to communicate spiritually, not to mention nurture your unborn child.

When worn or carried, crystals transmit peace; they give a sense of spiritual enlightenment that warms your heart like nothing you've ever felt. The vibrations they exude flow through your body the same as an electrical current. Once it settles into your life center and that of your unborn child, it will radiate nothing but love, strength, and wellness to both of you.

Using crystals while pregnant activates your child's intuitive feelings, making them more receptive to change and envisioning all things prosperous in the future. When your child gets older, they will feel more connected and in tune with the world around them. A happy and emotionally stable womb experience will bring forth a human being who is not afraid to secure a well-balanced future.

If you decide to use crystals during your pregnancy, it's important to remember that their energy will be a part of your child's growth and development while in utero. During this time, the baby will get used to these wonderful energies and will seek and crave them out of the womb. When the time comes to put your baby down to sleep, place a crystal inside a sock or something similar and hide it in their crib. The sock protects your baby from swallowing the crystal, and they will feel the peaceful energies that have been a part of their development for the past forty weeks. In turn, they will feel snuggly and safe just as they did while in the womb.

Throughout this book, I will suggest one or more crystals for each week of your pregnancy. If you feel connected to a particular crystal, then feel free to use it.

Remember, it is all about you, what you feel, and what makes you most comfortable. You may even find a new crystal you can connect with, one that you will eventually treasure.

Choosing a Crystal

There are numerous ways to select your preferred crystal, but everyone experiences their energies differently. The best way to do this is by looking at them to find the one that attracts you the most. It doesn't matter if the crystal is the same size as your little fingernail or one that fits perfectly in the palm of your hand. It's the one that inexplicably beckons you to take it home with you.

Crystals exude energy, but they also absorb positive or negative energies. This is why it's best to cleanse them before you make them a part of your etheric energy, your home, or your baby. There are many ways to cleanse them, and it's something you'll need to do each week before using that week's crystal. The simplest way to do it is to immerse the crystal in a glass of water, add a tablespoon of salt, and leave it outside for the night.

After your crystal is cleansed, you'll need to program it. Each week I will guide you how to maximize a particular crystal's essence. You'll also use positive visualization to merge the crystal's energy with yours and that of your growing baby. So hold the crystal tight after you cleanse it. Visualize the weekly suggestion for a better outcome and then use as suggested.

Music

The chakras have a specific music note that resonates within each one of us, like those of a musical instrument. When these centers are balanced, they hum within you to resonate spiritual awareness. Once this is accomplished, you can find yourself more in tune with your body, your mind, your emotions, and those around you.

Music ignites emotions to a crescendo of recollection that nothing else can ever match. It retrieves memories faster than taste and smell. A melody can attach itself to your music memory bank for life. By listening to a song that was relevant to a time in your life, it can take you back years and trigger those events, even decades later.

I am a firm believer in listening to music during pregnancy. It not only makes a bond—a connection with your unborn child—but it also holds that connection for many decades to come. Listening to music also gives the baby a peaceful womb experience. And if the mother is having a good pregnancy, not only physically but also emotionally, then the baby she carries within her womb could do no better.

There is no particular genre to play to your unborn child. Use the music you or your partner enjoy and relax with. Amniotic fluid is a good conductor of sound, so there's no need to listen to loud music. Just embrace the flow of the music as it wraps around you. While it does, hold your tummy and gently tap it with the rhythm of the song. You will feel the baby settle within you or stir with the beat, enjoying the melody and the enjoyment it brings to you.

I suggest wearing a jingle bell–like necklace while pregnant. These bells are also known as Harmony Balls and are easily found online. These tiny little bells clear the space around you from negative energy. Also, during the pregnancy, the baby will get used to its sound within the womb and the relaxing effects it brings. After birth, the baby will immediately recognize the sound and remember the comfort of the womb and, most importantly, you as that jingle bearer; in turn, the baby will settle quicker, feeling safe and very much loved with the bell-like sound they know all too well.

Still, I encourage you to play music throughout your pregnancy. Have the house vibrating with the sounds that bring you pleasure, joy, and relaxation. Music can stimulate your spiritual growth and bring comfort to the baby. Throughout the weeks I will guide you through meditations using music in the background. Select the music you relate to beforehand to get you in the mood for enlightenment.

In your child's future, you may find that not only do they remember the melody, the drum beat, and the string or piano section, but they may make a connection with some of the styles you liked, even adding them to their future playlists. There is no better feeling than your child enjoying the music you grew up with.

Color

The world is a collage of color that is constantly roaming with our emotions. Everything is filled with colors, some clear and bright, others shadowed with darkness and even sadness. We choose the colors we vibrate to and we repel those we absolutely hate, but each color has a physical and emotional purpose whether we like it or not. Our bodies need their energy to liven our existence, enhance our moods, and even heal our physical bodies.

Our homes are tastefully decorated with a color theme. Children are often dressed according to gender. Advertising and color go hand-in-hand. Company logos get bigger and brighter due to color consultants who specialize in the art of attraction and allurement of customers.

Any given color can make peace within our body and nourish our emotions and even our material needs. The chakras have designated colors within their depths, but this doesn't mean we stop using the other colors of the spectrum. How could we not when they richly complement the seven chakras? Unlike music that vibrates through our bodies, colors flow like silent radio waves, connecting our bodies with their life force.

Visualize whatever color is suggested each week and spread it throughout your body. See the color connect with your blood vessels and flow it and its energy throughout your body to your baby. You can achieve this by wearing the suggested color or displaying the color in any form you wish. You can even use a colored pencil to draw on a sheet of white paper to bring that color energy to your weekly space.

Color seeps through the skin like water in the sand. Let's say you've been feeling a little unsettled about your pregnancy. By wearing blue, a soothing cool color, you'll notice the unsettling feelings you've been having will dissipate. This goes for all the colors of the spectrum, as each color has a meaning and place in your emotional state of being.

Focusing on a color could be beneficial for your blood pressure, the emotional pregnancy roller coaster, and the health and emotional well-being of your baby. I will guide you to a particular color according to the baby's growth and where you are in your pregnancy. This doesn't mean you can't wear or use a color that attracts you. Pregnancy has a way of choosing the colors you wear or have around your home. I am certain the baby cocooned in your womb has something to do with it. This is why you may feel an attraction to a color you never particularly liked before. Your baby seeks the vibrational essence to grow and develop within the womb and is comforted when that particular color's vibration is felt.

Quick Color Summary for Your Pregnancy

Black: Protective
Blue: Calming
Green: Forgiving
Orange: Creative
Pink: Loving and Understanding
Purple: Spiritually Aware and Peaceful
Red: Strengthening
White: Spiritual
Yellow: Intuitive

Candles

We are often oblivious to candles' magnetic strength and therapeutic effects. Just as baths connect to the water element and crystals connect to the earth, the flame of a candle is linked to the fire element. It is the courageous spirit within each one of us, the soul of our inner strength and courage. Mankind has been lighting candles as far back as 200 BCE to see in the dark. Now we light candles for ambiance, relaxation, and to keep from using fluorescent light. We tend to light them when the chores of the day are done or after dinner to relax and reflect.

A candle's glow can relieve the stressors of the day and is a great way to communicate with your baby and spirit. It is a sight to behold when you dim the lights and see the flame of your candle flickering around the room. How could you not relax and feel surrounded by love, peace, and hope?

Apart from candles' soothing relaxation empowerment, they also have a spiritual connection to your oneness with the universe. If you give a candle's flame purpose as suggested throughout this book, the candle will light the way and give you peace and courage throughout this journey.

Every week throughout this book, there are going to be candles and a purpose to their flame for that week.

Light your candles with thought and spirit. Give the flame the purpose per the suggestion for that particular week. Give them your full attention, visualizing your intent and the outcome while connecting to the fire element's strength and resolve.

The candles will be a different color each week, sometimes two colors to connect with the oneness of your spiritual self and that of your baby. Use tapered candles when needed. If you can't find the colored candle you need, use a white candle and use things like colored plates, tablecloths, or even ribbons at the bottom of the candle of the color you need. You can also light tea lights, waiting until the wax is melted before mixing food dye with a toothpick to blend the food dye and melted wax.

Dig up all the candleholders you have around the house or borrow some for the duration of your pregnancy. When you see the light of the candle and remember the reason for it being there, it will warm your spirit and connect you emotionally and spiritually to your bundle.

Baths

Water encompasses the emotions and the waterworks of our existence. Water can take away negativity just as quickly as a river flows, bringing hope and optimism.

There is a reason we seek places near the ocean or look for the biggest resort pool to spend our vacations. It's because we need water. We yearn for it, crave it, and above all, we want to submerge in it to become a part of it. We want to feel the weightlessness of our bodies and silence the outside world just as we experienced in our own mother's womb. We want to feel that same protection. We want that buoyancy in our life. We want the cushion the water offers, not only physically but emotionally as well.

When we were in the womb, we knew peace and felt protected. We developed in a substance that could be classified as liquid gold, something that is very valuable to the life growing and developing within it. This is how the water element governs our life, not only spiritually but physically. We can't survive without it.

The amniotic fluid is your baby's lifeline, just as the umbilical cord and placenta are. And it's the best protective cushion your baby will ever have. This magical fluid is constantly circulating in and out of your baby's body, bursting with electrolytes, proteins, and minerals that are needed for the development of your child.

Having a bath while pregnant is a magical experience. A bath is great to soothe aches and pains. It relaxes the muscles and brings peace of mind to the soul, but most important, it is time to connect with your baby who is settled nicely in their own magical tonic. By embracing the water element, you connect and embrace the life growing within you to exist in the outside world with emotional stability, wisdom, and empathy.

I will suggest safe things to add to your bath that help you connect and tune in to your baby's frequency. An oil's energy, a flower, or even a dash from your herb rack can penetrate your skin on a spiritual level to relax you and bring you more in tune with the water that holds your baby's life in its depth.

You want your child to make good choices due to a happy and selfless womb experience. By using the water element through a bath, your child will know when to express their emotions, when to hold them, or when to freely let them go when they are older.

Things to remember while pregnant:

a) Make sure you always have someone to help you in and out of the tub.

b) The water should be lukewarm, never hot.

c) Have a non-slip mat so you can sit without sliding down.

d) Above all—enjoy!!

Caution: Make sure there is always a non-slip mat in your bathtub and shower. Have someone help you in and out of the tub for your own safety, especially during your third trimester.

Essential Oils

Essential oils have been around since ancient Egyptian times, possibly even longer. These essences are all-natural, carefully extracted from plants, herbs, and flowers. Due to the extraction processes, their healing and therapeutic properties make them stronger than the original plant.

These magical oils can make your home smell wonderful when used on your oil burner or diffuser. Not only do they make your home smell great, but they bring the flora kingdom right to your doorstep. These oils have the power to make you feel happy, emotionally settled, and comfortable within your own skin. Their therapeutic capabilities are endless, including soothing headaches, aching muscles, and nausea, and their essence carries charming magical qualities.

These oils are connected to the air element—the element of creativity, intelligence, and communication. By breathing in and anointing their essence (or massaging, when safe) while your baby grows and develops, you can start to affirm your baby's intuitive future. By using the oils, you breathe in their connection to the universe. And when you use essential oils for a specific intent, that intent will transfer to the growth and development of your baby on an emotional level. Look at it like your child is going to school, a baby in-utero school of emotional well-being, safety, and intuition.

When you use essential oils, you will find inner peace and you will be loyal to your pregnancy and the child you carry. You will relax quicker and you will be mindful of the things that upset you. Just by breathing in their scent for a specified purpose, you will find appeasement within you and focus on what is right in your life and not what is wrong.

While you are pregnant, there are certain essential oils that are not safe to use. I will NOT be including these in the weekly Mindful sections, especially in the first trimester, as some oils can add to your nausea. Check with your medical provider should you have any concerns, and always make sure your oils are essential and not synthetic.

If you have any of the essential oils listed in the caution list that follows, it's best to put them in a box and tuck it away in a dark, cool place until after your pregnancy. Be sure to look at their expiration dates before using them again, but you'll be surprised at how long their shelf life is.

I will also give you a list of the essential oils you will need at the beginning of each trimester to have at the ready for the coming weeks. Keep in mind, pure essential oils can be a little pricy. If cost is an issue, check with your friends to see if you can borrow an oil for that week. If you can't get your hands on the essential oil for that particular week, make lavender your substitute.

Caution

Oils to avoid unless supervised by a medical practitioner or an aroma therapist consultant.

- Basil
- Cedarwood
- Cinnamon
- Clary sage
- Clove
- Cypress
- Fennel
- Hyssop
- Jasmine
- Juniper
- Lemongrass
- Myrrh
- Parsley
- Pennyroyal
- Peppermint
- Rosemary

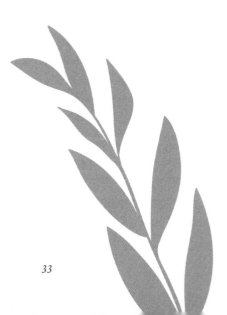

- Sweet marjoram
- Thyme

Flowers

Bach flower remedies have been around since the early 1900s. Edward Bach, the founder, believed the petal of a flower or plant held physical and emotional properties. He was so adamant that he found a holistic approach to their essence, which is still practiced today. There is also the folklore that surrounds flowers and their color to consider. Back in the 1800s, people took great care when choosing flowers for the home or social gatherings. When given, they expressed emotions and could break, fix, or start a new relationship. Over the years the folklore of flowers has diminished except for a few, which still remain true to their meaning.

The beauty of a flower awakens two of our senses: smell and sight. Some flowers are not as eye-pleasing as others, but their scent is wonderful. There are also those that are spectacularly beautiful and have no scent. Don't be fooled; they are just as potent with or without scent.

While you're pregnant, your focus is totally on the baby. At times, unwarranted concerns creep in without you knowing or wanting them. Your baby constantly develops and grows, and so do your hormones and emotions, which can magnify at the slightest nudge. These concerns sometimes outweigh the warm fuzzies of pregnancy, but flowers can turn those worrisome thoughts away. Let flowers be a focal point during your pregnancy to help you relax and enjoy the weeks until the end of your gestation. Their essence is calming and nurturing. Their colors will brighten your senses. They can help you release your worries and let peace of mind embrace you every time you walk past them. They will be a reminder that all is well and as it should be.

So bring a bunch of flowers home every week during your pregnancy. At the end of each week, take one bud from the bunch, place it in a dark place until completely dried, and then place it inside a brown paper bag. At the end of your pregnancy, you should have close to forty dried flowers. When you bring your baby home, take them out and pull the petals apart until all the petals are in front of you. Place them in a muslin bag and keep them with your baby's other keepsakes as a reminder of your beautiful pregnancy.

If you are unable to obtain the flowers suggested for that week because they are out of season or sold out, don't stress about it. If this happens, you can bring their energies to your home by drawing a picture of the flowers with colored pencils, crayons, or watercolors. While you draw the flower, visualize the energy it brings to that particular week of your pregnancy. Not only is this a relaxing and a spiritual exercise, but emotional art therapy for your soul.

Mindful Allies

Meditation

Meditation is a state of being and of thoughtful awareness. When we meditate, we don't focus on the external world but on the world within us. It's the world where we overthink and stress and where we constantly play reruns on everything that has happened, will happen, or could happen. We can't help ourselves. We all do it. And guess what happens when we do? We feed the frenzy and our minds never have a vacation from our thoughts and worries.

That's why it's so important to give our minds a rest, especially when pregnant. If we rest our bodies when we're tired, then why can't we do the same with our minds when we are worried or stressed? I see our minds as the mother ship that controls every single emotional response and every nerve ending in our bodies. It never shuts down, even while we sleep.

Meditating while pregnant helps calm your mind from the day or from any worries you may have. By holding on to the awareness you attain while meditating, you will be able to communicate with your baby and strengthen your child's growth, all while feeling reassured that all is as it should be.

There are more ways to clear the mind than meditation. There are also spiritual boosts such as nature walks, visiting friends and family, and going shopping for the baby. These spiritual boosts clear the mind while keeping you focused on an intent that is enjoyable and fun. In turn, you will feel more relaxed and happier that you have gotten out of the house and done something that is not mundane or a chore.

Meditation is a practice that you will benefit from even after the birth of the baby. Meditating around the same time every day gets you into a habit. Meditation helps to conquer your day, leaving you more rested, less stressed, and able to function more efficiently and calmly through the days of your pregnancy.

Visualizations

Visualization is a conscious daydreaming practice that activates the mind. The visualization practice can manifest what we want, what we need, or what we dream about. When we visualize, we create a guided imagery of our desires. The emotions we feel while visualizing can make a desire come to fruition. We can accomplish this by picturing or sensing a desire like watching a movie or reading a book. The good thing about this book or movie is you are the creator and you alone can visualize the ending to make it happen.

Perhaps you need a more reliable car when the baby is born, but you can't see a way to get one. Your finances may not allow it, or you may be putting money away for the expenses when the baby is born. Do not lose hope. You can visualize the car as if you already own it. Visualize yourself driving it, parking it, and putting the baby in the car seat. It only takes a few minutes and you can apply it to everything you wish or need. When the car eventuates, it could be in the form of a bargain, a swap, or even a gift. Knowing you have the power to will that dream or need into existence, the possibilities are endless. You are the director of your life and you can make it just as you want it to be.

Conducting positive visualizations while pregnant can aid you in visualizing the health and growth of your baby. You can visualize a happy and content child, or an adult that is positive and sure of where they are heading without emotional blockages or despair. You can also visualize yourself as a good mother and being fair in all things concerning your child's future.

There is no place positive visualization can't take you. You just have to see it, feel it, and know that you are seeing the possible future, the future you want to have with your child. Every time you think about the baby, visualize health and happiness. See your baby growing happy and healthy within you. Visualize a happy future for your child and let visualization be a part of your active future dreams while pregnant.

Affirmations

Affirmations are positive phrases you repeat to yourself daily, sometimes a few times a day, to manifest a positive outcome. Affirmations are a way to block negative thoughts from your mind by replacing them with positive ones. By repeating an affirmation that describes how you want to feel and be, you will change the way you act and think about yourself on an emotional level and become more open to positive possibilities.

Affirmations are easy and they become second nature once you get the hang of it. An affirmation gives you control so your mind doesn't take you where you don't want it go, like thinking negatively or catastrophizing events before they happen.

If you tell yourself when you wake up, *Gosh, I hate my job,* then your day becomes a flurry of negative events you have no control over, all brought on by a single negative thought. If you hate your job, then do something about it. Change the way you feel about your position or start looking for another job by telling yourself, *Until the perfect job comes my way, I will do the best I can with the one I already have.*

Affirmations help you stay positive and in control of your pregnancy even when you go into labor. Positive affirmations are a great tool to keep you positive, stay in control, and deal with daily events without stress taking over, like when friends talk about their hardships through their gestation or their own experiences with labor. No two women are the same. We all experience pregnancy and labor differently and you must not take on their experiences.

Affirming that all is well and as it should be does wonders for your pregnant state of being. Repetition is the key to a positive outcome and should be done on a daily basis—morning, noon, and night. You can write it down and place it on your bathroom mirror, your computer desktop, or even wrap a hair band on one of your fingers. These become reminders to say your affirmations when you see them.

I will give you an affirmation for each of the forty weeks throughout your pregnancy. Say it as many times as you can throughout the day to bring that positivity to you and your baby. As you get closer to delivering, the affirmations will ease you toward the upcoming labor. They will give you strength and self-esteem. Remember, you are running the show with your birthing team, loving partner, or whomever you choose to be in the delivery room with you.

I am strong, I accept the challenge
before me with ease, comfort,
and, above all, with love.

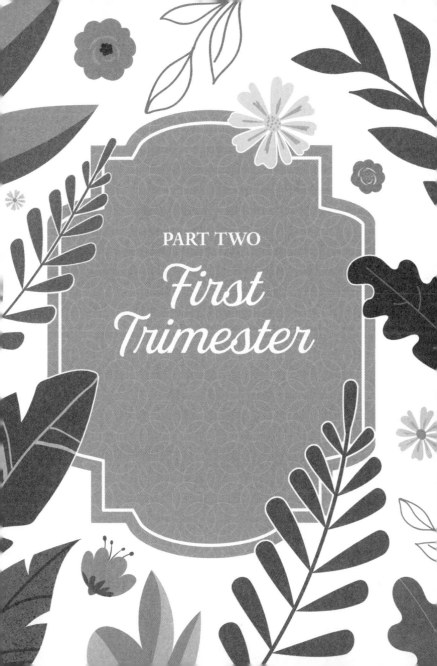

PART TWO

First Trimester

Tools Needed

Flowers

Geraniums

Birds-of-Paradise

Lilies—White

Carnations—Pink

Daffodils

Bunch of Flowers—Your
Choice

Chrysanthemums—White

Daisy—Red

Crystals

Carnelian Agate

Moonstone

Rose Quartz

Blue Lace Agate

Green Calcite

Red Jasper

Citrine

Clear Quartz

Amazonite

Red Jasper

Colors

Orange

Blue

White

Green

Yellow

Purple

White

Pink

Essential Oils

Clary Sage

Chamomile

Ginger

Lavender

Spearmint

Lemon

Bergamot

Ylang-ylang

Baths

Epsom Salts
Red Food Dye
Bay Leaves
Rose Petals
Lemon
Mandarin
Yellow Food Dye
Pineapple Juice
Coconut Water
Orange Food Dye
Spray Bottle
Orange Rinds

Candles

Yellow
Pink
White
Blue
Purple
Green
Red
Orange

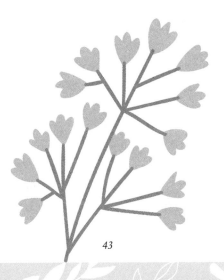

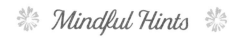

❋ *Mindful Hints* ❋

Conception

If you're not pregnant and picked up this book wanting a spiritual and mindful experience from the onset of your pregnancy, then Mindful Conception is for you.

Now that you've decided to have a baby, you likely wanted to conceive yesterday. Every time that thought creeps into your mind, remind yourself that over the years you've been telling yourself, *I don't want to get pregnant.* Now here you are, wanting it to be "now."

Once a woman has her first period and becomes sexually active, she typically guards herself against pregnancy. This not wanting to get pregnant tattoos itself on the back of a woman's mind every time she takes the pill or uses another type of contraception. Without you even knowing, this becomes an affirmation of not wanting to get pregnant.

The first thing you need to do is to erase this harmless affirmation you've unknowingly committed yourself to. Now replace it with a positive affirmation: *I want to be pregnant and I will get pregnant.* See yourself pregnant. Tell yourself and your body that the time is now and that you're ready to be a mother. Let the maternal essence reside within you. Let it engulf your body with positive thoughts, visualizations, and affirmations.

Keep in mind that some women conceive right away; others may take months to do so, or need a little medical help along the way. If it doesn't happen immediately, be kind to yourself and the woman you are and the mother you want to be. But above all—do not blame yourself and stay positive as you go through the conception process.

Below is a list of Mindful Hints to help you to stay positive along the way.

Bodily

- Make sure you exercise regularly to keep fit and to reduce stress.
- Eat a stable diet of healthy foods, including:
  - ~ Greens
  - ~ Fruit
  - ~ Salmon
  - ~ Berries
  - ~ Oysters (natural Viagra, filled with zinc for men)
- Take prenatal vitamins to support regular ovulation and a healthy uterine lining that is full of folic acid.
- Stop smoking and excessive alcohol intake.
- Get plenty of sleep and rest.

- Maintain a positive attitude.
- Do not get discouraged.
- Use a safe sexual lubricant that does not have spermicides.

Male partners should ensure they are also eating right. Vitamins such as zinc, selenium, vitamin A, vitamin C, and vitamin E are very important for sperm support. Fatty acids improve sperm life span.

Holistically

- Get acupuncture treatments.
- Enroll in a yoga class.
- Consult with a naturopath.
- Schedule a reflexology appointment.
- Use essential oils (inhale, burn, add to your bath, or dilute for massaging).
    - ~ Clary sage (corrects hormone imbalances and increases libido—female). *This oil is not to be used after conception.*
    - ~ Sandalwood and rose (increases libido—male)
    - ~ Frankincense oil (increases sperm count)
    - ~ Lavender (increases relaxation and regulates menstrual cycle)
    - ~ Patchouli (increases libido)

- Schedule a hypnotherapy session.
- Meditate regularly.
- Begin using positive affirmations, such as:
  - *My reproductive organs are sound and healthy.*
  - *I can and will create a new life.*
  - *I can feel the essence of my baby around me and within me.*
  - Never say, *If I conceive,* but rather, *When I conceive.*
- Engage in positive visualization (feel pregnant and see the growth around your tummy).
- Schedule a massage for relaxation.

Enchanting

- Use crystals (carry them with you or place them under your pillow).
  - Tiger eye, carnelian, and red jasper (together)
  - Moonstone
  - Rose quartz
  - Aquamarine
  - Turquoise
- Eat Brazil nuts (for male fertility).
- Drink lemon myrtle tea (for fertility, but not after conception).

- Seek spiritual guidance.
- The moon is associated with fertility, so try meditating with the moon as a focus.
- The Earth is grounding, so walk barefoot while digging your heels into the dirt. Visualize the Earth's strength within your womb to aid conception.
- Burn yellow and white candles next to each other.

The Tales of Worldly Grandmothers

- Bring a pair of yellow baby booties into your home.
- Do not wear earrings until after conception.
- Obtain a cloth diaper and pin it with large white baby pins as you would around a baby.
- Tie an orange ribbon around your stomach.
- Pin a white baby pin within your clothes (this is a way to tell the world you are ready for new life).
- Eat lots of bananas to increase sperm count (male).
- Eat carrot seeds to boost fertility (male and female).
- Eat figs (male and female).
- Put flowers in your house, including:
  - ~ Daffodils (in the bedroom)
  - ~ Geraniums (potted plant in the house or bedroom)

- Draw a bunch of green grapes and place it under your pillow.
- Use poppy seeds (put a handful in an orange drawstring bag and carry it with you to boost fertility).
- Have sex at sunrise.
- Have sex at a certain time to determine the gender:
  ~ Sex in autumn for a boy
  ~ Sex on a full moon for a girl

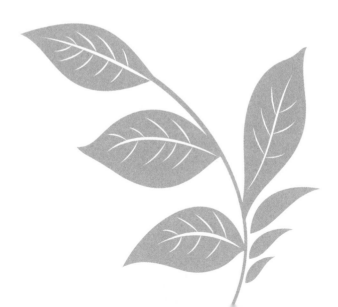

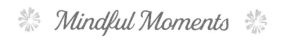

Mindful Moments

The Journal

Try to keep a journal throughout your pregnancy. The power of pen and paper can be a miraculous tool for expressing our deepest feelings. There is a sense of freedom when we write down how we feel. It's as if by writing it down we let go of whatever is bothering us, or we cherish the experience forever.

When looking for a journal, find one that is bright and beautiful, just like you want your pregnancy to be. Try to find one with pockets so you can slip keep things in it that are significant to your pregnancy. If you can't find one, get creative and make your own pregnancy journal. This may make it more meaningful and keep your focus throughout your pregnancy.

Get some colored pencils, make a cover, and use bright paper throughout. Section it with the first, second, and third trimester. Within each trimester, add personal notes and talk about your partner and how they are dealing with the pregnancy. Measure and weigh yourself so you can look back on it. Take notes on your highs and lows, what's bothering you, and how you handled it or how you plan to handle it. Count the kicks each day and when your baby is most active. Is it after certain foods or hot or cold drinks?

Also make note of the things that made you cry or laugh. Jot everything down, adding pages should you need to. Don't forget to keep special mementos such as ultrasound pictures and pictures of your rounded belly. You can even write small notes of encouragement to yourself. You can write baby name ideas, their meanings, and underline the one that feels right and why you chose it. Write down your fears and joys about being pregnant. Don't forget your cravings and the way people responded to the announcement—and of course your partner's reaction.

Make this journal your confidant throughout your pregnancy. It's nice to look back at the pregnancy and not depend on memories, which fade over time. But your journal will not. Later in life you may want to share it with your daughter, daughter-in-law, or even granddaughter. You may want to flick through the pages when you're in the mood or when you're next pregnant to get you excited to start journal number two, three, or even four.

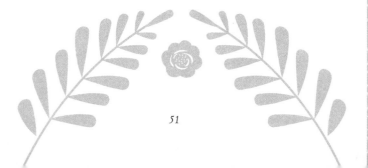

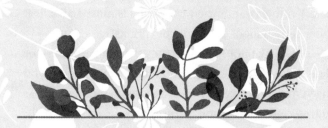

Weeks 1, 2, and 3

I am ready to be a mother
and nourish the essence
of what it entitles.

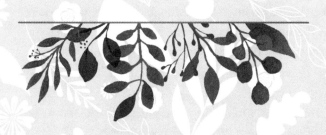

A date that you will be asked over and again when you conceive is the last day of your period. Write it down somewhere because this date starts the countdown to your pregnancy. Even if you haven't conceived yet, this is officially the first day of your pregnancy, as conception happens around two weeks from that day.

If you haven't had a medical checkup prior to conceiving, now is be a good time to do so with your partner. You will be asked questions about your health and both of your family histories. If your doctor has any concerns, he or she will bring them to your attention and conduct further needed tests. If your doctor is happy there are no underlying issues, then you have a green light to start this miraculous journey.

Flowers—Geraniums

If they are in season, find a potted bunch of Geraniums and placed them in your room. Geraniums carry the Goddess energy and fertility screams from their essence.

Crystals—Moonstone

For the next couple of weeks, carry a moonstone crystal with you. It will aid with conception. It can be in the form of a necklace, ring, or even a bracelet. It doesn't matter—as long as it's with you at all times.

What do you think your baby will look like? Is it a boy or girl? See yourself breastfeeding, holding, and cradling your baby.

There is one important thing you must keep in mind: Do not get discouraged. There are women I call *Fertile Myrtles*. They conceive on their first try. If it happens for you within the first or second try, then join the Fertile Myrtles. If it doesn't—don't despair. If you've been trying for a while, talk to your family doctor for guidance. It could just be a matter of timing, but in this day and age, there are many avenues and options you can take to help the odds.

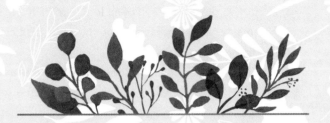

Week 4

I welcome the opportunity
to nourish life.

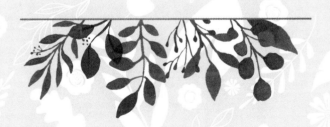

Baby—The embryo is now secured in the uterus. The tiny cell divides into two sections; one section will become the embryo and the other the center that will nourish the baby throughout your entire pregnancy.

Mother—When the fertilized egg attaches itself to the uterine wall, it signals the body to release a hormone called chorionic gonadotropin, which is traceable in the urine and confirms your pregnancy.

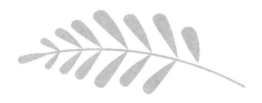

Flowers—Birds-of-Paradise

Birds-of-paradise are protective and vigilant flowers. They can also symbolize the joy of new beginnings whether it's your first, second, or third journey into pregnancy.

Crystal—Rose Quartz

Rose quartz opens the heart chakra that enables you to give love to the life that is now growing within you. Keep it close to your heart or in your bra, as it promotes healing, compassion, and forgiveness. Rose quartz enables hidden sensitivity, rather than acting with logic, because there's nothing logical about being pregnant—it's a miracle.

Color—Blue

During this week, your emotions are heightened due to the wonderful news of your pregnancy. Blue is soothing and protective. Blue pledges endurance, just as the sky is blue, and commits to your pregnancy by banishing any fears you may have.

Chakra—Root

The root chakra is, in a sense, in mild shock at this time. There is a foreign body attached to your life center. The root chakra is the survival instinct within each one of us. Not knowing if you're going to get through the next forty weeks and do the right thing for your growing bundle may make you feel uncertain and outright scared. Don't be, because what you're feeling is normal. By repeating the below affirmation as many times as you can during this week, you will ease the tension within the root chakra to manifest balance within all the life centers.

I am the warrior, the strength, and the peace my baby needs.

Essential Oil—Chamomile

Chamomile soothes and calms the emotions racing through your mind during this time. It will help you look forward to the weeks ahead. It will ease your stress and insecurities, bringing about peace and comfort to your soul. Start with a drop on your oil burner. If the smell doesn't bother you, keep adding drops until the scent is right and pleasant for you.

Bath

For the next two to three weeks, it is advisable to add Epsom salts to your lukewarm bath. These salts ease muscle pain as they relax the muscles. When your muscles are relaxed, you will be too. These salts will also get rid of any negativity and doubts you may have about not doing the right thing throughout your pregnancy.

Candles—White

There is nothing more beautiful than a single white candle burning and communicating with Spirit. White is the color of purity and honor. This week is all about adjusting to the fact that you are expecting and it will help you to communicate your deepest fears to Spirit.

Meditation

This week is all about attachment and for the cell to stay connected to the uterus. Play a song that comforts you, preferably something without vocals so you can concentrate on your intent. It is not every day that you find out you're pregnant, so play something that's true to the way you feel about your pregnancy. Remember, the song you play today will always remind you of when you found out you were pregnant. Dim the lights and light the white candle. Lie down, get comfortable, and put a pillow under your knees for comfort. Place the rose quartz crystal on your heart so you can send loving vibrations to the beautiful cells growing within you. Do not think scientifically, but as a mother-to-be. Visualize this tiny group of cells holding on to your uterine wall, happy to be there, snug in its casing while taking form as the person they'll one day be.

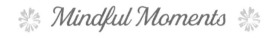
Mindful Moments

Broadcasting to Loved Ones

It may have taken you months, even a year, to conceive. Relish this moment. Feel your heart beating happily within your chest at the realization that you are going to have a baby and become a mother. Hold on tight, because this is an emotional ride that will last your lifetime.

If this was an unplanned pregnancy, take a deep breath and let the news sink in. Take your time, because there are decisions and planning to put into place. People usually tell their families soon after they find out, but typically not acquaintances or their place of employment until the twelfth week.

The first person to tell is your partner, unless they were present when you took the pregnancy test. If they were not, find a place where you know you won't be disturbed. Make sure you have their total attention. You can also come up with something fun to break the news. This can be enjoyable whether they were not expecting it or if the pregnancy was planned.

Don't forget to write their reaction in your journal.

Telling your close friends, parents, brothers, and sisters can be fun, especially if it's their first grandchild, niece, or nephew. If they are not expecting it, it can be a wonderful experience for everyone. Make it fun and something they will remember and share with their friends and the rest of the family when you're ready to tell the world of your pregnancy.

If this is your second or third pregnancy, telling your other children can be very memorable. I've heard of a woman who read a book to her small child about a mother telling her little boy she was going to have a baby. Another woman baked cupcakes and wrote "big brother" on one, and "little sister" on another. Older children can be a little harder, but they do come around. Friends of mine gave their fifteen-year-old daughter a rattle and let her guess its significance. When she did, she was ecstatic when she realized what it stood for.

Feel free to consult other people on how they broke the news to their children and family members. Start planning on how to do it. Think about telling the family about your pregnancy like it was a Christmas present and the baby was the gift. This gift has no monetary value but an emotional one that will last many lifetimes.

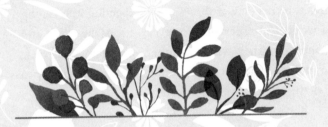

Week 5

I rejoice in knowing
I'm to be a mother.

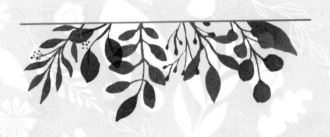

Baby—This week, the cell resembles a tadpole and is about the size of a poppy seed. The placenta has also started to develop. There are hints of black dots that will become eyes in the upcoming weeks. The arms and legs are but tiny buds ready to sprout. What is to become your child's heart is also taking shape.

Mother—Your metabolism will be slightly elevated. There are no signs that you are pregnant, but without your knowing, changes to your hormones, skin, and uterus are taking place.

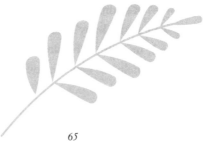

Spiritual Boost

Take a walk in a place filled with nature such as a park, a botanical garden, or even a small area filled with trees. Use your iPod or phone to find a song that relaxes you, something instrumental that moves your soul. If it's winter, bundle up and don't let the cold stop you. You'll still be able to find things in nature that are full of life. Visualize your womb just as strong and ready to support the life growing within you.

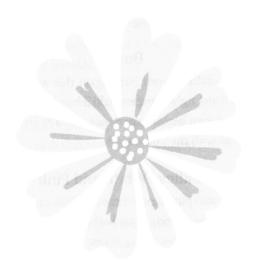

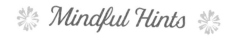

Mindful Hints

Partner Readiness

Not so long ago, men were left out of the birthing experience. It was considered taboo at one time. It was very rare that a man wanted to participate in the birthing process. Even doctors and midwives didn't like them anywhere near the mother, so as to not stress her out. We've come a long way from this thinking, as it's now widely accepted and expected for the father to show his support.

Keep your partner up to date with all your prenatal care. Better still, have them come with you to all the ultrasounds and prenatal care appointments with medical providers, midwives, or doulas so they don't feel left out. People tend to forget the partners in all the prenatal activities, but they are definitely an integral part of your pregnancy and the birthing process and should be included.

Male partners need lists. Not a honey-do list, but a list of the roles they will be participating in throughout the pregnancy and birth. Then they know what is expected of them. There is no use in getting angry with your partner if he doesn't know that his smelly socks can now actually make you dry heave, or that you may not be able to wash your feet soon and may need his assistance. If you don't tell him, don't expect him to know.

There is nothing more rewarding than preparing for this journey together with the person you love. You can make your partner feel included and let them know that their participation in all things is needed and most important, wanted, and valued. This makes the journey so much simpler, happier, and positive for both of you. Your partner may not be giving birth, but they will be by your side cheering you on until you reach the finish line.

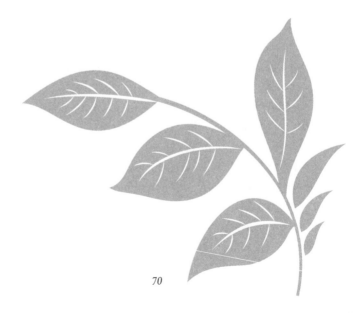

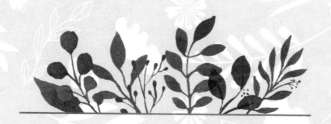

Week 6

The light growing within me
is developing, strong, and healthy.

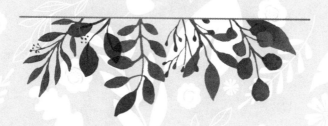

Baby—Your baby looks like a tiny shrimp. The cells have just about doubled in length. The changes taking place are happening fast. Vital organs have started to develop. There are two prominent black dots present, which will become your baby's eyes in the next weeks.

Mother—You may feel a little lightheaded as your blood vessels relax. The skin of your nipples gets a bit darker and the mucus plug starts protecting the uterus from infection until is expelled when labor begins.

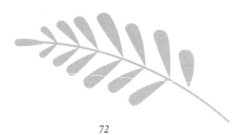

Flowers—White Lilies

Lilies not only intoxicate the senses, but they are very protective and bring harmony to the home. They can also cheer you up if you are concerned about the upcoming weeks.

Crystal—Blue Lace Agate

At this time, blue lace agate can strengthen your relationship with your partner. It will also cool any anger you may feel before it can surface by keeping it by your bedside or carrying it with you.

Color—Blue

Blue is a relaxing color that you should take advantage of as much as you can while pregnant. It not only relaxes you, but it can be very beneficial to help you express yourself with your medical team and to open communications with the baby while in the womb.

Chakra—Crown

Concentrate on the crown chakra this week. You can find it at the top of your head. This chakra is the psychic energy that communicates on a spiritual level between you and your baby. The affirmation below will affirm the communication needed between you and the baby. Say it as many times as you can during this week. You can also use this affirmation at any time throughout your pregnancy.

*I communicate with the life within me
and the life within me communicates with me.*

Essential Oil—Chamomile

Once again, use chamomile oil in your diffuser or burner to keep your mind stress-free. This oil will also protect your thoughts from turning negative, no matter what you read or see in relation to pregnancy.

Bath

Stick to Epsom salts again this week but add a whole thinly sliced orange to the bath. You'll find the essence of an orange will harmonize your hormones and lift your mood.

Candles—Blue

A blue candle this week will help you feel connected. When you light it, watch the flame as it steadies in front of your eyes to bring peace and joy to your working week. If you don't work, then do it to balance the inner peace inside your home.

Meditation

Find a comfortable place where you will not be disturbed. Have your candle close, your crystal in your hand, and the flowers nearby so you can see and smell them. Play a song or melody that you wish to share with the baby, something you think the baby will like when they're in their teens.

Close your eyes and find your inner peace. It doesn't matter where it is, as long as you can find it. In this meditation, think about what's happening in your womb. Visualize your child's heart disease-free and beating happily and steadily.

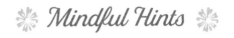
Mindful Hints

Staying Active and Fit

Finding time to exercise should be on the top of your pregnancy wellness list. Thirty minutes a day of moderate exercise can strengthen your pregnancy physically and mentally, not to mention give you more energy throughout the day and throughout your pregnancy.

Exercising is also a way to blow off steam. It releases chemicals to improve your mood, makes you feel better about doing something for yourself, and most important, it reduces stress. Exercise can also help with the baby brain, as it improves memory by pumping blood to your brain to help you think clearly and positively.

A brisk daily walk should be a priority, together with yoga to stretch your aching muscles and to stabilize emotions that can run rampant throughout your pregnancy. There are also stationary bikes and light weights you can utilize for core muscle and physical strength. You can do swimming, which is another preferred exercise to tone muscles while pregnant. As to now introducing a CrossFit or kickboxing class or contact sport, this is not advisable. You should check with your medical team for your safety as well as the baby's, even if you are already heavy into any sports or physical exercises.

Mindful Tools

- Carry a clear quartz or a garnet crystal to give you the motivation needed to get out there and do what you know is beneficial for you and the baby.
- Say this affirmation when you lack motivation.
  *My body in motion is healthy
  and vital for a healthy and mindful pregnancy.*

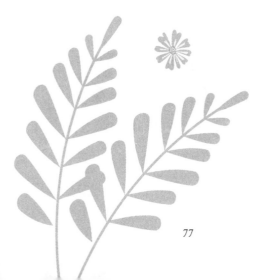

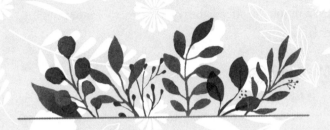

Week 7

With every breath I take
and with every single beat of my heart,
I give love to my baby.

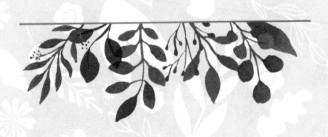

Baby—The embryo is the size of a blueberry. All major organs are developing to their full potential but not yet functional. The growth of brain cells is extraordinary and constant. The digestive system and lungs are forming. The embryo is covered with a layer of skin to protect it from infections while in the womb.

Mother—Even if you physically can't tell you are pregnant, your uterus is expanding. Your breasts tend to look and feel slightly larger and you may wonder how much bigger and darker your nipples can get. Your skin is going through some changes as well. It may be a little blotchy due to all the hormonal changes you are experiencing.

Visualize what you think your child will look like. What color hair will he inherit or what color eyes will she have? Will he look like you or your partner or a paternal or maternal grandparent? Will he be tall or short? Will she be kind and loving?

Visualize your healthy and happy future child smiling up at you, seeking your hand for guidance. Give yourself a pat on the back at the great job you or you and your partner have done to have such an emotionally stable and loving child.

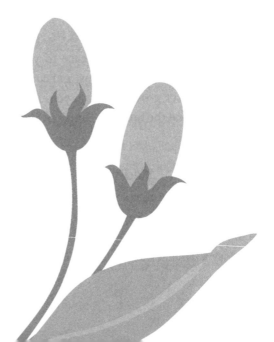

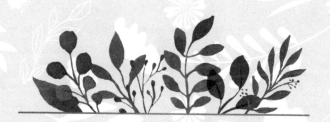

Week 8

Feel safe, little one.
You are perfect, loved, and cherished.

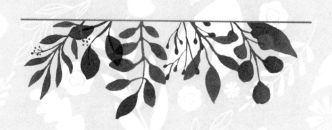

Baby—About this time, the baby is roughly the size of a raspberry. There are tiny jerking movements you are not aware of taking place within your womb. Your baby starts looking less shrimp-like and more humanoid right about now. The baby seeks nourishment from your physical and spiritual strength to grow and develop until the end of its cycle.

Mother—You have probably started to feel nauseous—morning sickness is no fun! Some foods are less desirable than others. Some scents can be offensive, and mood swings can invade your personality. You can also find yourself getting a bit more tired throughout the day.

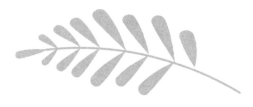

Flowers—Daffodils

Daffodils represent happiness and well-being. They are filled with love and kindness. This flower symbolizes the commitment you are making to your growing baby. It's all about rebirth and new beginnings.

Crystal—Red Jasper

Red jasper is a protective and grounding stone. This crystal will enhance your connection to the life that is growing within you. Red jasper stabilizes your hormones and the growth tissue of your baby and strengthens survival within your womb. You can't go wrong with this crystal close to you.

Color—Green

Green is the color of nature, which is always in a constant cycle of rebirth—as is the baby you carry. Wear green this week to strengthen the growth within your womb.

Chakra—Root

The first trimester is all about survival. It's about making your growing baby feel safe and secure within your womb. When you think about your baby, put your hands on your lower abdomen and say the affirmation below as many times as you can throughout the week.

You are safe and you are loved.

Essential Oil—Lavender

Burn lavender in your oil burner to calm the daily stressors this week. Lavender is soothing, calming, and eases stress. It brings peace to your pregnancy and love to the home. Start with a drop at first and see if you can tolerate the scent. If you can, you can add extra drops until you get the scent that's just right for you.

Bath

A warm bath will help you relax by letting go of the things you don't want in your pregnancy. Add a few rose petals to your bath to make you feel love. Add a sliced lemon to bring joy, along with one or two cups of Epsom salts. Sink in and relax, allowing your growing baby to get comfortable within your womb while feeling safe and loved.

Candles—Pink

This week's candle is pink to express love and understanding. It will give you comfort and surround you with acceptance and love. If you feel loved and secure, so will your unborn child.

Meditation

Find your meditation space and a music piece without vocals so you can concentrate on the intent you wish to manifest. Play a piece in C major. If you can't find one, play what makes your soul sing. A song or melody that touches your soul can do wonders for your physical and mental stability and can comfort your growing bundle.

Dim the lights and light the pink candle to communicate with Spirit. Burn the lavender oil on your burner; hold the red jasper in your hands. Have the flowers close by so you can see them and their yellow beaming strength and knowledge.

Now that you have created the scene, make sure no one disturbs this time with your unborn child. Lie where you are most comfortable. Make sure your feet are up and place a pillow under your knees for comfort.

Close your eyes, knowing you are in a safe environment. As long as you feel safe, so will the baby growing and taking shape within you. Visualize this tiny being, happy and content, enjoying the taking-shape process within you. Feel the connection between the two of you growing and settling in for the many weeks to come.

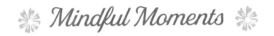

Mindful Moments

Bonding with Your Bundle

Some women take to pregnancy like ducks to water while others become cautious, especially if it wasn't a planned pregnancy. If you are one of these women, don't be hard on yourself. After the initial disbelief or shock wears off, you'll embrace the pregnancy as if you had planned it. The good thing about bonding with your baby is that you don't have to wait for the birth to do it; you can start from the onset of your pregnancy.

Be yourself while you hold and nurture life. Just like you sit and talk with your friends and family over a cup of tea or coffee, you can do the same with your baby—but not in public if you're on your own. People might think you're crazy! But you can silently or mentally communicate with the baby. Tell the baby stories about you growing up, your first memories of your mother and father, your grandparents, and what you used to do as a child. Tell the baby about your school days and everything that has left you warm and fuzzy over the years. Tell the baby how you met your husband or partner and the courtship that resulted in your current condition. *Keep it G-rated, girls*. The baby will hear these stories and connect with the emotion when you retell these stories later in life. Share the happy and emotionally heartfelt chapters of your life.

While pregnant, a woman unknowingly rubs her tummy. Is this action instinctual? Or is it simply that you are aware of the life growing within you? It's not going to be uncommon for you to feel movement or kicks when you rub your tummy later in the pregnancy. The baby will respond to and anticipate your loving, reassuring touch.

I know this may sound weird, but think of your tummy as a mobile phone. Every time you touch it you call your baby to let him or her know that you are there through the magical process of nurturing life. With a simple touch to your tummy and soothing words, you let the baby know you care or want the baby's attention. The emotion in your voice mimics feelings as if you were caressing your tummy. Even later in your pregnancy, you may feel the baby pressed hard against your bladder. Give your tummy a little poke and tell the baby, *Hey, cheeky monkey, please scoot over.*

You may, at times, be pleasantly surprised when they do.

There are more ways to connect with your baby than these simple tummy tactics and throughout this book you will be doing just that. They say a happy, peaceful, and loving womb experience creates a positive and well-adjusted child in the future, so let's do this!

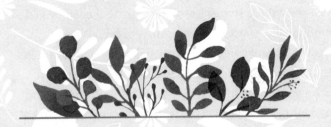

Week 9

Love radiates through
me and my baby.

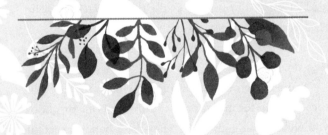

Baby—The baby's still growing at a fast rate and it's now about the size of a stuffed olive. It graduates from an embryo to a fetus this week. The webbed fingers have started to separate. The nose has started to protrude. The mouth and lips develop, as do the wrists, which can bend the tiniest bit. There are also ears now, which haven't taken their rightful place on the head yet. Even the digestive system is ready, but not yet functional.

Mother—Your body is now the mother ship. Your respiratory system adapts to help with the demand your body now needs. Nausea has really set in and you're not feeling like your chipper self, but sluggish.

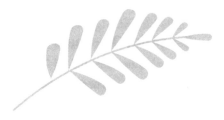

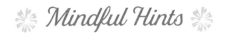

Mindful Hints

Work and Pregnancy

If you work during your pregnancy, you may find it more challenging than before you were pregnant. The high volume of work, which never bothered you before, could bother you in the upcoming weeks. Your boss may seem a little more demanding. Requesting time off for your prenatal appointments or because you feel sick may give you a sense of unease. This is normal, so don't let it get to you.

Concentrating on your job is what's going to get you through these coming weeks. You know your job better than anyone. If you have clients, then you know which ones are easy or hard to deal with, so prepare accordingly. After discovering you're pregnant, it may take time to get back into the swing of things at work. But don't worry—you'll be fine once you've adjusted to the wonderful news.

Keep your mind active, keep an appointment book, prioritize, and don't let things get too busy. Space your appointments so you can have a cup of herbal tea in between to settle your senses. Take time-outs, don't overdo it, and abide by your medical practitioner's advice on what your limits are if you have a physical or demanding job.

Remember, you need to look after yourself and keeping your stress levels low should be a priority. Find a trusted coworker to discuss any work concerns you have, or bounce ideas off them when needed.

Here are a few things you can do to make work a little easier and more peaceful.

- Use an oil burner or diffuser to diffuse lavender and bergamot to keep you relaxed and brighten your day.

- Keep an amethyst crystal at your desk to relieve stress and onyx to absorb negative energy.

- Drink lots of water to flush your kidneys. This also gives you an excuse to walk to the bathroom to take the pressure off your back.

- Bring flowers to brighten up your work environment, even if it's just one.

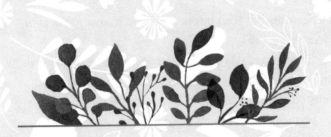

Week 10

My baby's heartbeats
are strong and healthy.

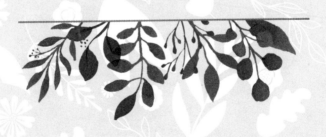

Baby—The baby is approximately the size of a prune. The placenta is working hard to feed the baby the nutrients it needs. Even if you still can't feel any movement, the baby is very active. The neck is functional, and the ears are in place. The heart has four little chambers and its heartbeats are circulating blood throughout the baby's tiny body.

Mother—Your uterus starts to move up the pelvis, which means less pressure on your bladder. The uterus also starts to accommodate your growing bundle by stretching as the baby grows. Flatulence may make itself known and dreams can be very vivid.

Look at your upcoming obligations, especially in the third trimester. See if you have any scheduled trips that need to be changed or rearranged according to your due date.

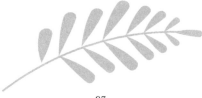

Flower—White Chrysanthemums

Find a large bunch of white chrysanthemums that have lots of petals. These white flowers convey trust and honesty to your unborn child, letting them know you will always be there as a mother and future friend.

Crystal—Clear Quartz

This crystal will aid with the detoxification of your body. When you detox yourself, you detox your baby. Place it by your bedside for peaceful sleep and dreams.

Color—Purple

Get a pair of purple pajamas or nightshirt. The purple reassures the baby that even if you're not talking or moving as you do in the daytime, you are still there, breathing and nurturing. The color purple can also bring sleep to your sleep-deprived world.

Chakra—The Crown

The crown chakra encompasses oneness with the universe. The affirmation below is an excellent way to communicate with your guides, angels, and even your baby's assigned soul.

I seek peace with all there is
and for my baby and his/her future self.

Essential Oil—Lemon

Last week I suggested you use spearmint. If it's helped with your nausea, please keep using it. If it hasn't, try lemon essential oil. Its antispasmodic properties can settle your stomach.

Bath

Instead of a soothing bath this week, treat yourself to a relaxing body massage. It will loosen all the tension from your body and the baby will benefit as well. Don't forget to tell the massage therapist you're pregnant to ensure they use safe essential oils.

Candles—Green

As discussed in previous weeks, green is the color of growth and prosperity. It also builds muscle tissue, which is perfect for the development of your baby. When the candle is lit, visualize your baby growing and getting stronger within your uterus.

Spiritual Boost

This week, take several walks and concentrate on the good things in life. Think about the things that have made you feel good over the years, as well as the things you want to achieve once the baby is born. Talk to your baby, tap your tummy, and let them know you are there and always will be. Include your partner and their accomplishments in your thoughts as well. You and your partner are not just emotionally connected. You're now physically connected as well.

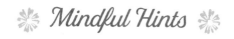

Mindful Hints

Stress and Pregnancy

You are more sensitive and aware of everything around you when you're pregnant. The sensitivity in every single nerve ending in your body is heightened. Your hormones pull you every which way while your body adjusts to the first trimester of your pregnancy, when you are most vulnerable.

You may have concerns about being pregnant. How can you not? You are going through amazing daily changes that have your head spinning, wondering how much more your body can stretch. Just thinking about it is enough to take you out of your comfort zone, not to mention the mysterious road ahead, especially if you're a first-time mother.

Your hormones are like the strings of a violin, played by a rookie. If that doesn't make you shudder, nothing will. The pull, the pluck, and the tightening to tune it is nerve-racking and it won't be silenced until you relax. You can do this by not letting daily stressors consume your pregnancy. Cutting down on stress will not only make it easier and healthier for you and the baby, but it also lets you enjoy your pregnancy while nurturing your child in the womb. Take time out. You aren't doing yourself favors by not doing so. There's always going to be some level of stress in your life, even when you're not pregnant, but you alone can control the level of stress you experience during your pregnancy.

When you're stressed, try some of the Mindful Hints below:

- Step back and breathe.
- Go for a walk. With every step, let go of the stress that binds you.
- Light a blue and a white candle in your home to calm your emotions.
- Flick the stress from your shoulders to let it go. There is no need to hold onto it, especially if it's out of your control.
- Carry an amethyst or a blue lace agate crystal to keep your stress at bay.
- Play songs you know relax you and remind you of happier times.
- Stay away from red and vibrant colors. Instead, wear soothing pastels to keep you calm.
- If a person causes you stress, stay away from them. If you're comfortable, discuss it with them. If it's someone at work, talk to your boss to see if they have suggestions to minimize conflict.
- Go to a meditation and relaxation class.

- Do something that makes you happy and you enjoy, like a hobby or something you've always wanted to try.
- Visit with friends and loved ones.
- Go out with girlfriends and drink a non-alcoholic beverage from a wine glass.
- Have a cup of peppermint tea to settle your tummy.
- To settle your mind from worry, carry the petals from a white rose in a blue drawstring bag.
- Add a few drops of lavender essential oil to a spray bottle filled with distilled water. Spray it around the house and on your clothes, but not on you during the first trimester.
- Place your hands on your sacral chakra, where your child is settled in your womb, and say:

> *This is not your stress but mine to deal with,*
> *and deal with it I will.*
> *Feel and know that you are loved,*
> *wanted, and cherished.*

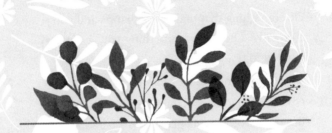

Week 11

I love being pregnant
and cherish every second
of this magical experience.

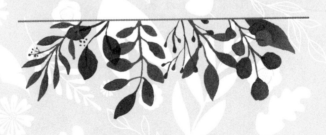

Baby—The baby is now the size of a lime and all sorts of wonderful things are happening. The left and right brain hemispheres are visible. The head is more rounded. The ears are neatly pinned where they should be. The umbilical cord is fully developed and feeds vital nutrients to the baby. All extremities are clearly visual and bent slightly.

Mother—You start to see the changes in your body as your clothes feel tighter, especially around your midsection. Your nausea could start to decrease, and your energy levels start to rise.

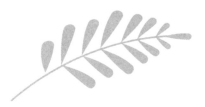

Flower—Planting

This week, plant something in your garden such as herbs, flowers, or a tree. If it's winter, bring an indoor plant into your home. You can watch it through the upcoming weeks to see how much it grows, just as your tummy will soon flourish.

Crystal—Amazonite

This crystal promotes spiritual healing and growth. It removes any negative doubts you encounter during this time. It will also help with morning sickness should you still have it.

Color / Chakra / Candles

The reason we crave a color is due to the baby. We also crave colors that help us absorb the energy our body needs through our chakras. By lighting a candle and eating foods of a particular color, you nourish the body with the spiritual color nutrient you and your baby need.

Incorporate these three Mindful Tools this week by picking a color that stands out above all others in the spectrum. Consult your baby and I assure you that one color will stand out. Let's say blue attracts you this week. Then wear mostly blue and burn blue candles this week.

As for the chakras, pay attention to the color of the foods you crave. Red foods are for energy, orange for self-confidence, yellow for an emotional pick-me-up, green for emotional stability, blue for self-expression, purple for spiritual enlightenment, and white for a connection to the universe. Every time you crave a vegetable or fruit, think of it as the color you and your baby need to balance a chakra.

I replenish what was freely given with love of color.

Essential Oil—Bergamot

This is a happy and refreshing oil to brighten your week. Burn bergamot essential oil in your oil burner or place a few drops in your diffuser. It will calm you and bring a content disposition to you and your baby.

Bath

Add a few drops of bergamot essential oil to your bath this week. If you are sensitive to the smell, try just one drop before adding more to get the right scent. The smell will bring a smile to your face when you sink into your bath. You can also add a few orange rinds, a few slices of lemons, and a few drops of yellow food dye.

Before you know it, you'll be in a magical, fruity cocktail that's positively divine and full of happiness.

Spiritual Boost

If you are able, make a mother-daughter date with your mom. If she's far away, plan to Skype or FaceTime. Talk to her about her pregnancy experiences over a cup of herbal tea. Ask her how your father took the news about her pregnancy with you or any siblings. Ask her how she faired with her pregnancy and tell her about yours.

If your mother has passed away or if you don't have a healthy relationship with your mother, talk to someone you are close to or regard as a mother. Ask her to share her experiences with you and you share yours with her.

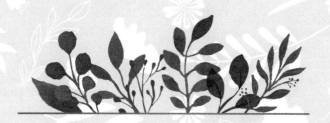

Week 12

I feel wonderful as I progress
through my pregnancy.

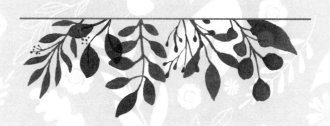

Baby—The baby is around the size of a plum right now. The baby peacefully floats in the amniotic fluid and has plenty of room to grow and mature. The eyes are closed, and the baby's muscle control is developing.

Mother—The unpleasant morning sickness you've been feeling may have started to fade, but in some women, it can last longer, and in others, it can last throughout the pregnancy. Around this week, your strength comes back and your energy levels lift as your hormones start to settle. Some women experience a heightened libido.

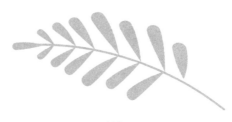

Flowers—Red Daisy

Bring playfulness back into your relationship now that you feel better and have more energy. A daisy's essence can increase sexual drive if your libido has plummeted, putting sex back on the table.

Crystal—Red Jasper

Red jasper purifies the blood and revitalizes the brain by improving mental acuity and finding hidden courage. Keep it close to you to balance your emotions.

Color—White and Pink

This week's colors are white and pink. White communicates with your spiritual beliefs and convictions and pink conveys the innocence in your heart. Together, these two, colors purify the magic tonic within the placenta your baby comfortably lives in.

Chakra

All your chakras are working overtime as your pregnancy progresses. They adjust to your emotions while making sure the life growing within you is happy and content. The affirmation below will help you stay grounded. Try saying it morning, noon, and night.

I breathe in light and exhale what I do not wish to hold on to by keeping grounded and true to my life source.

Essential Oil—Ylang-Ylang

This week's essential oil should be used during the meditation to focus on gratitude and express love.

Candles and Bath

Light a red and orange candle in your bathroom for strength and courage. Fill the tub and add Epsom salts to help relax any tense muscles. Add a cup of pineapple juice and a cup of coconut water before sinking into the bath. You may be close to telling your place of employment about your pregnancy and this can be a little daunting. This bath will settle your mind and help you focus on a positive outcome.

Meditation

Go to your quiet meditation place. Play relaxing music, something mellow and romantic. Hold the crystal in your hand and close your eyes. Relax until you feel centered and happy that no one will disturb you. Smell the sweetness of your essential oil in the background. Visualize a white light penetrating your womb that's filled with love and pureness.

Think about where your baby is in their growth cycle this week. The eyes are formed and yet the lids are still shut. Visualize your child seeing clearly with marked acuity. Visualize your child reading people in the future for what they are beyond the exterior and into their souls.

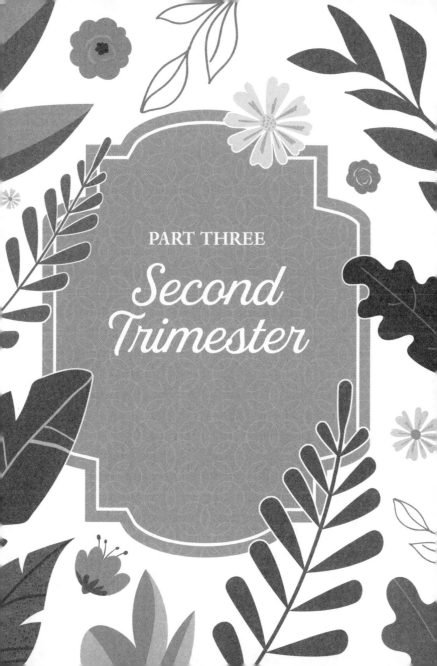

PART THREE

Second Trimester

Tools Needed

Flowers

Gerberas

Orchids—White

Basil—Bunch

Pansy

Roses—Mauve

Baby's Breath

Daisies

Lilies—Pink and White

Sunflowers

Gladiolus—Green or Yellow

Rosemary—Bunch

Persian Buttercups

Fennel—Bunch

Crystals

Aventurine

Amazonite

Citrine

Fluorite

Ametrine

Garnet

Unakite

Clear Quartz

Sodalite

Carnelian Agate

Moonstone

Rose Quartz

Colors

Yellow

Black

Blue

Pink

Green

Purple

Essential Oils

Neroli

Ginger

Rose Geranium

Geranium

Rose

Sandalwood

Lemon

Sweet Orange

Chamomile

Frankincense

Lavender

Patchouli

Baths

Coriander
Green Food Dye
Rose Petals
Wheat Germ Oil
Fennel
Thyme
Eucalyptus Leaves
Brown Sugar
Star Anise
Spray Bottle (100 ml)
Cinnamon Sticks
Goat Milk
Honey
Table Salt

Coconut Milk
Almond Oil
Aloe Vera Oil
Pineapple Juice
Blue Food Dye

Candles

Orange
Purple
White
Blue
Tea Lights
Green
Yellow
Pink

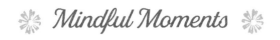
Mindful Moments

Telling the World and Your Place of Employment That You Are Pregnant

These days, couples typically don't share their pregnancy news until the twelfth week when they know all is as it should be. If you haven't divulged your status, plan to do it before they think you're getting fat instead of pregnant, as happened to me.

You'll be surprised at how happy people will be about the news. You might wonder why you waited so long to announce it. But there is one person that might make you anxious about sharing the news, and that's your boss. When you're ready to tell him or her, have a backup plan for your position while on maternity leave. You can suggest people they might place temporarily in your position, or perhaps your job can be divided among other team members while you're on leave. Your boss will appreciate that you thought about your position and the company while assuring them it can be accomplished.

Above all, be truthful to your employer; tell them if you're coming back and if you are, in what capacity. Whatever their response is, don't take it personally. Don't let company policy and ethics deter you from sharing your pregnancy news.

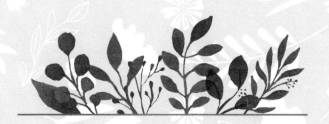

Week 13

I celebrate the beginning
of my second trimester.

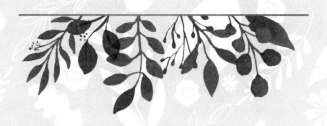

Baby—Your baby is the size of a peach and is in proportion as the trunk starts to lengthen. The hands and feet are no longer webbed. The vocal cords are forming, readying for crying outbursts once out of the womb. The baby is moving around easily and posing in all sorts of positions.

Mother—As your body volume increases, your skin will start to get that famous pregnancy glow. Your little bump can no longer be hidden, so show it off proudly as you carry the start of your future family.

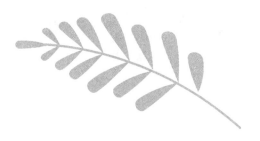

Flowers—Gerberas

There is no better way to celebrate the beginning of your second trimester than with a bunch of assorted colorful gerberas in your home to compliment the happiness and joy you feel.

Crystal—Aventurine

This is a crystal that has many faces, which is why I recommend keeping it close as a communication tool between you and your baby. Every time you see this crystal leading up to your delivery date, tap your tummy and say, *Hey darling, I'm here and I love you.*

Color—Yellow

Yellow is a happy color. Wear it this week to activate your baby's inner spiritual strength and brain capacity.

Chakra—Sacral

Concentrate on the sacral chakra the first week of your second trimester, which is exhilarating. This chakra is all about new experiences with a creative undertone for your baby. The below affirmation is filled with creative expression.

My child is a canvas ready to come to life.

Essential Oil—Neroli

Neroli deflects negative habits and thoughts when you burn it on your oil burner or diffuser. It also aids you to make a connection with your child. Breathe in its essence and think of nothing but a positive future for your sweet little bundle.

Bath

For this week's bath, add a few drops of lavender oil and two drops of green food dye and the leaves of a large bunch of coriander. This bath will relax you and steady the flow of oxygen through your body and the baby's body. Some old wives' tales say coriander can raise the brain activity of your growing baby.

Candle—Orange

Light an orange candle this week when meditating to connect with your baby.

Meditation

Go to your meditation space. Put your neroli oil in the diffuser or oil burner, hold onto your aventurine crystal, and light your candle. Place your flowers nearby. Play some enjoyable classical music that soothes your soul and your baby.

Look at your flowers and the radiance their essence brings. Then, close your eyes and take a deep breath to center your mind. See yourself as an invisible life force journeying through your body until you penetrate the placenta. When you do, take physical form and float next to your baby. Look at your baby's little body, eyes shut. The baby senses your presence and you both feel comforted.

Take your time and introduce yourself to your child as their mother. Tell them how much you love and care for them. Tell them you are always going to be there for them and that they will grow to be wise, strong, and smart. Tell them they will have a heart that will forever hold love and understanding.

After this meditation, you'll feel elevated knowing you travelled to your own womb to introduce yourself to your child.

How cool is that?

(Please feel free to make this journey as many times as you wish throughout the rest of your pregnancy.)

Week 14

My breathing has no limits
but that of the divine force.

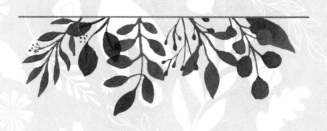

Baby—The baby is now about the size of a lemon. The umbilical cord is longer and thicker and passes oxygen, blood, and nutrients to the baby. If you are having a girl, the ovaries are being fine-tuned and she will be born with all the eggs she will ever have. Genitals are increasing visually.

Mother—You may have a stuffy nose caused by extra blood flow to the mucus membranes. You could start suffering from constipation and indigestion if you're not already. Remember to take your time when you eat and watch out for foods that produce gas. Expel gas when needed. You might find you can't help it. Don't feel bad about it; after all … you're pregnant.

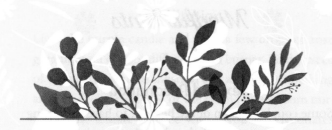

Week 15

My child will filter through
life's problems with ease and comfort.

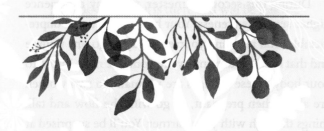

Baby—The baby is approximately the size of an orange. The kidneys are functioning, filtering blood and getting rid of the waste from the baby's body. There is eye movement. Messages from the baby's brain to the rest of the body travel fast and expediently through the baby's body.

Mother—You skin is glowing and your hair is fuller and glossier. You may even notice that your hair is not falling out as much as it has been. Your nails become stronger and you can't find anything wrong with the world. This is because you are sedated from the outside world due to your pregnancy, and this is a wonderful feeling. Enjoy it!

Flower—Bunch of Basil (Herb)

Bring a healthy bunch of basil into your home this week. Yes, basil. Display it as you would a bunch of flowers. The basil's essence is love and it brings abundance and prosperity into your home.

Crystal—Citrine

This crystal's strength and perception is like no other. It will aid your decision-making about the future and your baby's learning experience in the not-so-distant future. For best results, keep it close or under your pillow at night.

Color—Black

Wear a black ribbon around your right wrist this week. Every time you see it, think of something negative you want to get rid of. At the end of the week, cut the ribbon and throw it away, along with all the negativity it now possesses.

Chakra—Solar Plexus

The solar plexus is where you find your liver and kidneys. These two organs are filtering systems in our body. They filter bodily waste, but we also filter and dispose of our emotional waste through this chakra. The affirmation below is to help the baby filter emotional waste in the future with ease and comfort.

My child will breathe in daily challenges
and filter through them like a flowing stream.

Essential Oil—Rose Oil

This week, bring more love to your state of being with rose oil. Why not share these emotions with your partner? Use a few drops of rose oil in your oil burner or diffuser to convey your emotion. It will flow through your partner as well as through you and the baby.

Note: To minimize the cost of rose oil, you can use rose oil with a jojoba blend.

Bath

This week's bath is simple. Out of all the oils you've used thus far, find one that you made a connection with and use it in your bath. Add whatever else you want to use, like Epsom salts or a dash of wheat germ oil to relax your skin, making it silky and smooth. While in the bath, connect with your precious cargo, telling it you love it now and always.

Candles—White and Purple

This week, light a white candle and a purple candle. White is pure and purple is holy, just like how your pregnancy is progressing.

Meditation

This week, play something classical that warms your heart. Get comfortable in your meditation space. Look at the candle and the bunch of basil that is close by. Take a few deeps breaths of your rose oil to center your physical and spiritual self.

Visualize your child growing up with everyday challenges like school, friends, or relationships. See them unfold in a positive way. Do this while repeating to yourself: *There will be no problems my child cannot filter, there is no fear my child will not conquer, and there will be no emotional challenges my child cannot come to terms with.*

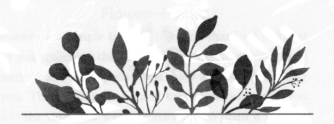

Week 16

My baby is growing strong, healthy, and wise.

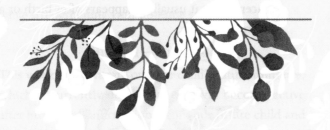

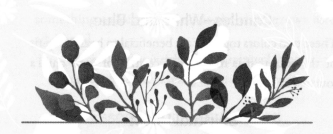

Week 17

I love my partner
and my partner loves me
and our baby.

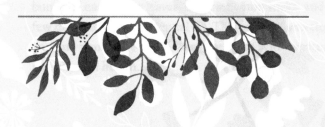

Baby—The baby is about the size of a pear. Its organs are clearly visible now. The baby is curled with legs and knees bent. The skin is transparent. The baby's heart is now regulated by the brain and beating steadily and faster than yours.

Mother—Your heart is working a little overtime; your blood pressure could be slightly higher than before you got pregnant. Internal and external body changes continue to occur. Have a checkup with your dentist if you experience bleeding gums. If you have dry eyes, consult with your optometrist to relieve the symptoms. While you're there, have your eyes checked for any other discomfort you might have.

Flower—Mauve Roses

Around this time in your pregnancy, you might need a little TLC. Purple or lavender roses are a great pick-me-up to find the self-esteem you may have lost during your pregnancy thus far.

Crystal—Rose Quartz

This crystal is a combatant of self-doubt and insecurities, should you have them. If you don't have those feelings, carry it with you to expand the etheric field around your body to express the love you have for your baby.

Colors—Pink and Yellow

Your partner may be feeling a little left out around this time. Keep in mind that your partner wants to understand the things you're going through in your pregnancy. By burning these two candles together, you can share the connection you have with your baby with your partner.

Chakra—Root

You need to be grounded now more than ever. There are a lot of things that will occur during the next few weeks as you approach the halfway mark. You need to affirm that you're ready for the next part of the journey. The affirmation below will help get you there.

I am grounded and open to what is yet
to unfold and welcome the experience.

Essential Oil—Sweet Orange

Start with a drop of this oil and see how you feel. I find it a little strong, but try it, even if it's just a drop. Sweet orange helps you navigate new experiences and can help you through emotional turmoil during your pregnancy.

Bath / Candles

Do something fun in your bath this week. Invite your partner into the tub while you both still fit. Light about ten tea light candles before filling the tub. Add a drop of lavender oil in each tea light after some of the wax has melted. Then pull each petal off one of the mauve roses and add them to the bath with four drops of rose oil and two drops of ylang-ylang.

Relax, enjoy each other's company, and talk about the life growing within you that you both get to share in the not-so-distant future.

Spiritual Boost

Take a walk somewhere with water—the beach, a lake, a river, or around a stream. This will tune in your emotions to your child. As you walk, make sure you take note of what you see. Notice everything around you and tell yourself what you're seeing so you can share it with your baby.

If you see a tree you like, describe it in your mind's eye and how it makes you feel. By doing this, it will help you stay grounded and tune in to nature. It also nurtures your baby with love and the beauty of what they will soon see.

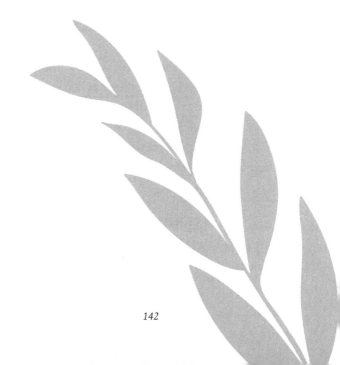

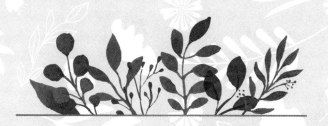

Week 18

I felt my baby move and I am enlightened by the experience.

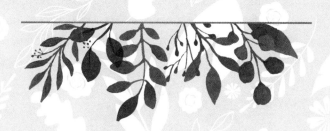

Baby—The baby is about the size of a bell pepper and resembles a little person now. Facial features are well formed; finger and toe prints have started to develop. The baby is active and happy floating in the womb without a care in the world.

Mother—You may have felt the baby move before, but noticeable movements typically begin between week 18 to week 23. The experience is surreal! It may feel like a flutter or butterflies in your tummy and no … it isn't gas. This is known as the quickening, and as the pregnancy progresses, these butterflies become kicks. Closer to the end of your pregnancy they are measured and hard.

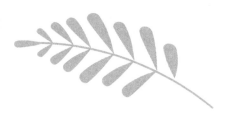

Flower—Baby's Breath

Celebrations are at hand—you felt your baby move! Bring a bunch of baby's breath home and display the tiny flowers that represent love and innocence.

Crystal—Fluorite

During pregnancy, your bones and teeth may suffer as the baby absorbs calcium from your body. A fluorite crystal can aid your bones and gums. After this week, try to keep this crystal on top of your night table or under your pillow until the birth and even when breastfeeding.

Color—Yellow

Yellow energizes muscles into motion, which the baby needs. This color is intuitive, active, and warming. Your baby is maturing quickly, and a little extra yellow will not go astray now that you're feeling its movements.

Chakra—Throat

Sometimes it's hard to express what you feel, and it can be even harder when you're pregnant. It's not because you don't want to, but because you can't identify what you're feeling. This is because there is so much going on with your body that you can't express it. Your vocal cords will not cooperate. You may even get a bit of a sore throat because you may not be expressing how you feel. Say the affirmation below to help express yourself.

I express what I feel freely
and so will my baby when wise and older.

Essential Oil—Chamomile

If you feel a little restless before going to sleep, burn chamomile to help you seek slumber, or have a nice cup of chamomile tea before bed.

Bath

This week's bath is what I call the Egyptian Goddess. Fill the tub. Take a green candle up to your bath. Add two cups of goat milk and a cup of honey to your bath—warm the honey so it will be easy to dissolve in the water. Add a few daisies or lilies to your bath and a few teaspoons of table salt. Sink in and find your inner goddess and when you do, your baby can't help but benefit from the effects of this bath's energy.

Candles—Green

Lighting a green candle can level out your emotional state of mind this week. It will bring clarity to your mind and positive and loving thoughts to the baby. Green is also a growth color, which the baby needs to keep growing healthy and strong.

Spiritual Boost

This week, get your girlfriends together and go out on the town. Go out to dinner and have fun, laugh, maybe even go dancing! Just because you're pregnant doesn't mean you can't dance. After all, dancing is good for your physical state of being; just make sure no one knocks you over. Your girlfriends have your back because that's what girlfriends do.

You have no excuse not to have a drink, because there are plenty of non-alcoholic drinks out there. You may feel a little tired closer to the end of the night, but you'll know when you've had enough and it's time to head home.

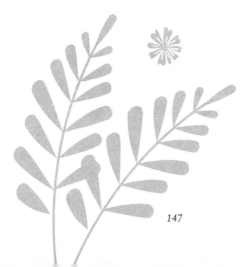

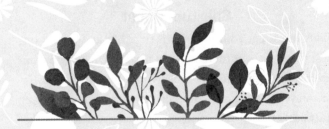

Week 19

My baby can hear me
and recognizes the sound
of my muffled voice in the womb.

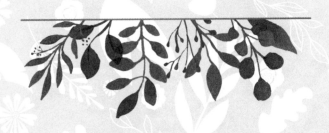

Baby—The baby is approximately the size of a mango according to the baby fruit-and-vegetable charts. The baby's sense of sight, sound, taste, touch, and smell are developing. A fine growth of hair now covers the baby. The baby will spend most of its time asleep when not active in its space.

Mother—Weight gain accelerates; your breasts keep getting larger. Your body temperature warms so you feel hot all the time. Wear cotton to help your skin breathe through these crazy, wonderful times. Make sure you keep all your prenatal appointments; they will increase even more during your third trimester. Empty your bladder often to avoid urinary tract infections, especially after sex.

Flower—Sunflowers

What a great way to bring sunshine into your home. There is nothing these positive flowers can't do or celebrate. Enjoy these yellow-orange blossoms to awaken the intuition of the one that resides within your womb.

Crystal—Ametrine

Ametrine is a crystal that focuses on the abundance you want to have. It also strengthens your relationship with your partner and child. It brings in an abundance of joy and happiness to your world. This is a crystal you should always have in your home.

Color—Mother-to-Be to Pick

If you have colored pencils, find a nice sunny spot and draw whatever comes to mind on a blank piece of paper. When you finish, look at your masterpiece. You'll notice there might be one or two colors you didn't use or used very little. This means that those chakras are well balanced, not to mention you and your baby have enjoyed a quiet pastime.

Chakra—Solar Plexus

Most of your baby's chakras have the essence of what they will be one day. They are flowers waiting to bloom. The affirmation that follows will help you concentrate on the baby's solar plexus, which is just below its little chest. It strengthens your baby's resolve, helping it to be forewarned and able to judge people before they have time to jeopardize your child's emotional sensors.

My child's intuition grows fruitfully within my womb.

Essential Oil—Frankincense

This oil is not something you'll burn or diffuse for its smell, but for the essence it possesses. This oil is spiritual, healing, loving, and reduces stress and tension. This week, use this oil to open your spirit to let it know you are well and happy, as is your baby. Be ready to be rewarded with great happiness.

Bath—Mindful Shower

The night before or a few hours before your shower, add one drop of frankincense oil, half a teaspoon of brown sugar, a star anise, and a few petals of one of your sunflowers into a 100-milliliter spray bottle. Fill with water, shake gently, and let it sit. When it's time for your shower, spray its contents into your loofah, your washcloth, or whatever you use to wash. Gently run it over your body, especially on the areas that need soothing from aches and pains.

Let this magical essence bring health to any physical ailments you may be suffering from and let the water element take away the ailment down the drain. Keep spraying on the affected areas until empty and repeat whenever needed.

Candles—Yellow and Orange

These candles burned together awaken spirituality and psychic abilities. Use these two candles this week to find the person you were before you got pregnant and to see the person, the mother, or the friend you wish to be to your child.

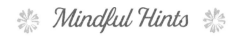

Mindful Hints

Gender Disappointment

There are some genetic tests you can do early in your pregnancy to determine the sex of the baby, but most women wait until week 19 or 20, when the gender of the baby can be clearly seen via an ultrasound—that is, if the baby's position allows it. When it's time, some couples choose to find out the sex of the baby while others don't. Some have a big gender reveal party with family and friends. Unfortunately, finding out the sex of the baby can be disappointing to some parents who are already set on a gender.

Some couples who already have two boys may be hoping for a girl or vice versa. Some want a child of each gender, knowing financially they can't have more than that. So, not getting the girl when you have a boy or two boys can be disappointing, especially to the mother-to-be.

Gender disappointment is a reality. Some women battle through this phase of pregnancy more than others. They may not talk about it, feeling guilty at feeling disappointed and not accepting the sex of another boy or girl. It can be disappointing on so many levels and can be hard to understand for those who may judge these women's emotions, seeing their disappointment as being ungrateful.

Unfortunately, these beautiful mothers beat themselves up about feeling discontented about the gender.

It's okay to feel disappointed and no, you are not a bad person and you won't be a bad mother. Talk to your partner to see if they feel the same way. Even if they do, they'll help you through it. Be sure to talk about it and don't shut yourself off. Talk to your medical provider and let them know how you feel, as they may offer some assistance. In the meantime, there are things you can do to let go of what's in your heart.

Have a good healing cry; get it out of your system and take a deep breath. Once you settle down after your cry, write down all your frustrations and disappointments, the reasons why you wanted a girl or boy, how it makes you feel, and the pros and cons of the gender you're having. Write down anything else that comes to mind. Don't keep anything in. You can even use capital letters to get out your frustrations on paper.

Once you're finished, wait about an hour and read it out loud. Somewhere deep within you a flicker of light may surface while acceptance warms your heart. Light the piece of paper on fire with a match in a fireproof container. Burn it until there's nothing left but ashes. Go outside and throw these ashes to the wind. As you do, see your baby, not the gender. See your baby that will forever be loved and cherished.

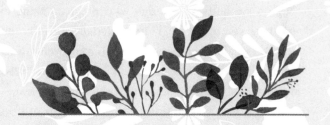

Week 20

Halfway Mark

I'm halfway through my pregnancy
and I love the way I look and feel;
I am beautiful.

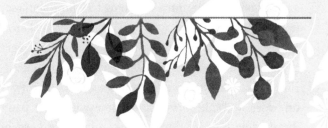

You are halfway through your pregnancy and by now you might feel better physically and emotionally. You've most likely gone through your twenty-week comprehensive ultrasound and confirmed the actual due date and the gender, if you wished.

These are exciting times. So many things to plan, so many things to put into place, and so many things to be grateful for at this stage of your pregnancy. Your baby is growing, and its nervous system begins to work more effectively, not to mention more actively. Your body warms and you feel hot all the time, more so in the summer months.

Your feet swell and you may feel a little tired, but exercise will help you through it. Exercise is a critical part of a healthy pregnancy and if you haven't continued with your exercise routine or the one given to you by your medical provider, get out there and start walking. If you don't want to go alone, ask your partner or a friend who doesn't mind listening to your pregnancy ups and downs.

Explore

This week, take time out for you. If you can, take a day off work and take some alone time with your baby. Bring some favorite flowers into your home, hold or wear your favorite crystal, and feel the comfort it brings you and the baby. Burn your oil burner or use your diffuser to conjure a blend that strikes your senses. But remember, don't make it overpowering, as your scent senses are still sensitive. Take a relaxing bath, use Epsom salts to relax your muscles, burn a candle by the bath, and tune in to who you are and who you want to be when your upcoming mother role takes possession of all your senses. Tell yourself over and over again:

> *Once I transition into the mother role,*
> *I will be the best mother my child*
> *would ever want to have.*

Take time to meditate this week and play music that relaxes you and warms your heart. Rub your tummy playfully and feel the essence of your child deep within you. Visualize the baby's lifeline, the umbilical cord supplying the much-needed oxygen to your baby that is as pure as sunlight. See your baby taking in the nutrients you provide, which are imperative for its growth and development.

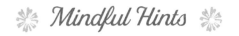

Mindful Hints

Baby Brain

"Baby brain" is the term referring to the minor memory mishaps pregnant women have throughout their pregnancy and sometimes after the baby's birth. Researchers have found that pregnant women have lower general cognitive functioning to those who are not, and it seems to affect the mother more in the last trimester.

The fog pregnant women experience is frustrating, to say the least. It makes us forget things we normally wouldn't forget, such as birthdays, our purse in a restaurant, or even a dinner engagement. Unfortunately, it does get worse if we give it too much importance and stress out about it. The fog is there and there's little we can do about it but be vigilant. The good news is that our cognitive functioning goes back to normal once our hormones level out after birth. So, don't think about it too much, but if it's impeding your everyday life, seek your medical practitioner's advice. Until your baby is born, there is little you can do about it, so try to go with the flow.

To help with this foggy feeling, write things down and have your work and home calendars up-to-date. Then refer to your lists and calendars to handle everyday issues and avoid missing appointments and important dates.

To lessen the fog, you can carry a fluorite or citrine crystal to enhance memory and strengthen your mind. You can also use grapefruit and lemon essential oils to keep your mind active and fresh. Burn them or place them in your diffuser for a pep of mental clarity.

Just remember, becoming a mother changes the way you think and prioritize things. Your mind may feel a little wacko and you might become absentminded during pregnancy. But this is just another temporary discomfort for the rewards that are yet to come.

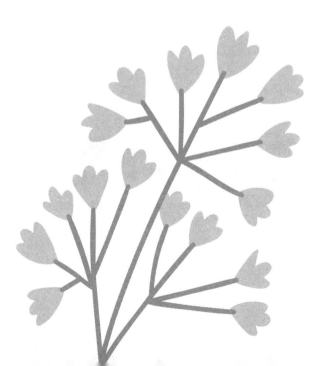

Week 21

My baby's lungs
are strong and developing daily.

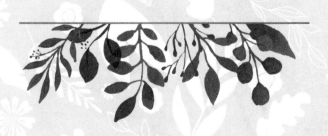

Baby—In the baby fruit-and-vegetable comparison guides, the baby should be about the size of a banana or pomegranate. This week is specifically dedicated to your baby's lungs. The stronger the lungs, the better it is for your baby if born prematurely.

Mother—If you have problems concentrating, eat more frequent and smaller meals. This will help keep you focus on the things that need doing and your digestive system will be grateful.

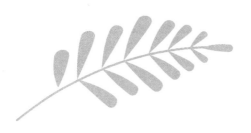

Flower—Green or Yellow Gladiolus

These flowers are all about never giving up and excellent to keep your baby's little lungs developing for the next couple of weeks of your pregnancy.

Crystal—Garnet

Garnet keeps organs healthy and functioning. Wear or keep a garnet in your bra this week. Every time you see it, visualize your baby's lungs strengthening in unison with your every breath.

Color—Green

This week, wear as much green as you can to strengthen your little one's lungs to carry the baby until its birth.

Chakra—Heart

The heart is the pump that gives life and enables us to breathe and connect with those we love. Fluid is pushed out of the lungs automatically. The baby practices breathing movements and when it does, the lungs grow strong. This is the perfect time to say the affirmation below out loud to make it so.

Every breath I take strengthens the lungs of my growing baby to breathe with gentle ease and comfort.

Essential Oil—Lemon

This week, use lemon essential oil for mental awareness. This essential oil helps with concentration and alertness. It will help you remember to stay on top of things without looking at a list.

Bath

This week, treat yourself to a massage. You're ready for another one to soothe all those little aches and pains that twinge, but most of all, relax.

Candle—Yellow and Green

These two colors will strengthen the baby's lungs when burned together, which is crucial at the halfway mark of your pregnancy.

Meditation

Let's start the next part of this journey by addressing the lungs during your meditation. Go to your quiet place again; play music that makes you comfortable and relaxed. Look at your beautiful gladiolus next to the yellow and green candles and smell the essential oil all around you. Take a deep breath and tune into the life force within you.

Visualize your baby's lungs rosy and pink. See these two tiny organs grow strong and healthy and see them strengthen through the next few weeks of your baby's development.

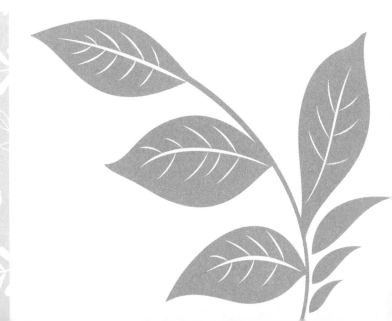

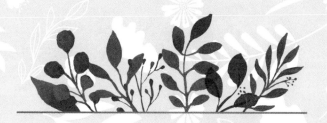

Week 22

I pass the beauty within me
to my unborn child.

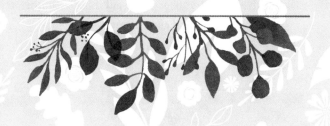

Baby—The baby may weigh around 15 ounces this week. Tiny nails have begun to emerge, and hair might start to appear on the scalp. The eyelashes and eyebrows are apparent. The baby can detect the difference between light and dark.

Mother—At times you may feel like there's a party in your tummy. The kicks are stronger, movements are weightier, and when the baby is still, you wonder if it's asleep or okay. You may feel itchy from dry skin and you may feel muscle aches and pains at the back of your legs. To aid this discomfort, try to stay as hydrated as you can.

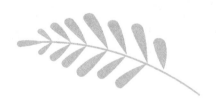

Flower—Bunch of Rosemary (Herb)

Display a bunch of rosemary as you would flowers. This herb is excellent for retaining your and the baby's physical awareness. It also stimulates hair growth, which is excellent at this stage of your baby's gestation.

Crystal—Unakite

Unakite aids with hair growth, something you want to wish upon your child while you hold this crystal, especially now that hair is starting to appear. You can also rub this crystal on your tummy for reassurance.

Color—Pink or Purple

These two colors are soothing and calming, which can help with your dry skin this week so you don't scratch too much. These colors can also help you relax your weary muscles and to sleep soundly.

Chakra—Crown

This week, concentrate on protecting and insulating your baby's future oneness with the universe. See your child connecting to the universal force, understanding its purpose and open to its function. Recite this meditation as often as you can this week to bring emotional comfort to the baby's future.

At this time my child is in a world of muffled silence,
comforted by the wholeness of a future,
open to all there is and what it will bring.

Essential Oil—Lavender

When you put this oil in your diffuser or oil burner, you will feel peace. Every time you breathe its essence, concentrate and feel your aches and pain soothe and relax.

Bath

This week, pamper your skin. Add two cups of coconut milk, a half-cup of almond oil, a few drops of lavender essential oil, and a half-cup of aloe vera carrier oil to your bath. Sink into your tub and let it gently soothe your dry skin. As you do, visualize your child's skin as soft and smooth as the water feels while you massage the bath water on your skin.

Caution: Have someone help you in and out of the tub, as it could be slippery. Ask them if they could clean the tub for you after you're done.

Candle—Orange

The color of this candle stimulates hair growth. Every time you light this candle this week, visualize your child's hair growing healthy and strong.

Mindful Look

At this time, it's a good idea to start thinking about who will look after the baby if you're going back to work after your maternity leave. If a family member has volunteered, that's great, but if not, you need to decide who is going to when the time comes. Make it a project you and your partner can do together. Make a spreadsheet with all the daycare centers around the area where you work or live. Visit them during the next few weeks and see what they have to offer to make an informed decision as to who is going to look after your precious little bundle.

You have plenty of time to choose, but sometimes a popular daycare may have a waiting list. If you want your child to attend a certain facility, it will help to start earlier rather than later.

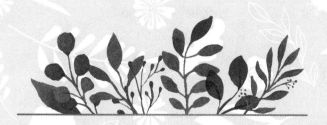

Week 23

This week, I am empowered
by my pregnancy.

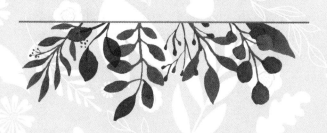

Baby—The baby is about the size of a grapefruit. Its skin is growing faster than its body. The baby can now hear loud noises and be startled by them. The baby becomes familiar with your voice, so talk as much as you can to your baby and sooth it with love.

Mother—There is a lot going on with you at this time, not only physically but emotionally as well. Your tummy is constantly growing and will keep doing so until the end of your pregnancy. Apart from all your aches and pains and discomfort, this is the best stage of your pregnancy, so relish the feeling. After you have the baby, you will miss those wonderful movements and kicks.

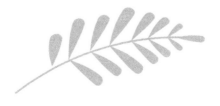

Flower—Persian Buttercups

These happy yellow flowers represent youth and childhood. Display them with a happy disposition while visualizing a happy childhood for your child in the not-so-distant future.

Crystal—Clear Quartz

This week, place three smooth (tumble stone) clear quartz in a one-liter bottle. Fill it up with water and place it in the fridge. Drink from this bottle as much as you can, as it will give you energy and ease aches and pains.

Color—Black

I know, I know … wearing black while pregnant may sound weird, but black is soothing and very protective. Black gives a sense of sincerity and strength. This week, wear black when you need strength to defy the things that are troubling you and protect you from others' negative thinking or your own.

Chakra—Throat

This week, project a positive tone in your voice when you speak. The baby is as attached to your emotions as you are. Now that the baby can hear your muffled voice, let it hear something gentle with the soothing affirmation below.

My words are but a sea of warmth
and love in my baby's ears.

Essential Oil—Patchouli

This ancient oil is nothing but generous with its essence. It brings peace and sexuality back into your world. You may not need it, as the hormones increase your libido daily, but if you've gone in the opposite direction, patchouli can guide you back to sexual awareness.

Bath

Use a few drops of patchouli oil in your bath if you need sexual awareness. If not, use lavender to pacify the urges if you want to do so. Add a few petals of your buttercups and a cup of Epsom salts. Sink in and feel the relaxation it brings to those tired muscles and deprived or exuberant urges.

Candle—White and Blue

This week, curve your uneasiness into hope and positive outcomes using these two colors. There are negative, insignificant thoughts that can creep into your mind that can start a war within you to destabilize your everyday being. These two colors can help you combat them and protect your mind.

Meditation

Close your eyes and settle nicely into your meditation space. Hold the clear quartz crystal in your hand. Keep your candles close and feel the essential oil and beautiful flowers fill your senses. Allow the music you chose for this meditation to soothe the stressors of the day. Take deep breaths and concentrate on your baby's hearing being sharp and acute for the rest of their life. Visualize your baby having excellent physical hearing as well as spiritual hearing as it tunes into the softness of your voice and the love it bears.

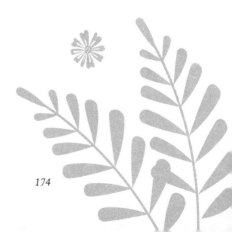

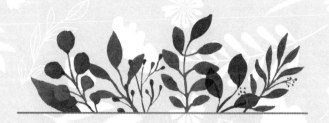

Week 24

I do not fear the unknown
but look forward to
what is yet to come.

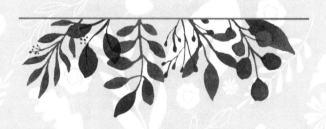

Baby—The baby is roughly the size of a piece of corn on the cob. It has also started to take control of its senses. The baby is even yawning and hiccupping. It has also developed sleeping patterns, which you have most likely noticed.

Mother—Your abdomen is expanding quickly and stretching to accommodate the baby pressing against your diaphragm. You may even feel breathless as the baby cuddles against your stomach area, which could lead to heartburn or acid reflux.

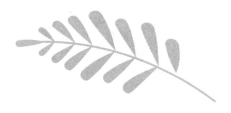

Flower—Fennel

Bring a fresh bunch of fennel into your home and display it like a bouquet of flowers. Visualize it bringing you health and healing energies, especially now, when you may start to feel uncomfortable.

Crystal—Sodalite

This crystal is great for balancing hormones while you hold or wear it. Its blue color and swirling white lines calm your emotions and focus on the feminine essence while soothing the subtle aches and pains of pregnancy.

Color—Pink

You could be feeling a little down about your weight gain or from your lack of energy. Pink alleviates the lack of self-esteem and gives your love-thyself motor a kick-start.

Chakra—Root

Expressing love to yourself is just as important as the love you express to your unborn child. Love your body while pregnant. There is little you can do to change the way you look, so love your body and go with the pregnancy flow. Affirm that you love being pregnant and don't let anyone tell you different.

I love my pregnant body and my pregnant body loves me.

Essential Oil—Ginger

Add a few drops of ginger essential oil to your oil burner or diffuser. This spicy aroma can have a positive effect on your endorphins and help with the way you feel about the way you look.

Caution: This essential oil is strong and spicy, so start with one drop at a time.

Bath

Add two cans of pineapple juice to your bath this week as well as a few drops of rose geranium essential oil for a sweet pick-me-up. This bath's intention is to make you happy and comfortable with the beautiful pregnant woman you are.

Candle—Pink

The flame of a pink candle is tender and peaceful and will bring loving energies to your heart and your baby's heart this week.

Spiritual Shopping Boost— Maternity Clothes

Wearing clothes that are too tight or baggy could be the reason why you may feel a little like an ugly duckling. These clothes may make you look like you've gained weight versus emphasizing your pregnancy.

Take your partner, mother, or girlfriend with you to shop for maternity clothes. Get yourself a few outfits, preferably ones you can also wear for a few weeks after you have the baby. Don't forget a good maternity bra, which you may need now. Be proud of that tummy. Show it off because you carry priceless cargo inside and that deserves recognition.

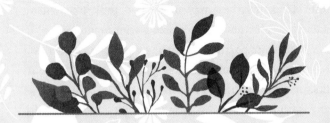

Week 25

I am loving the mother I am
and the mother I will be.

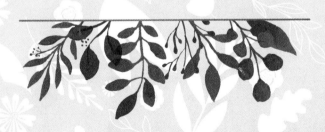

Baby—The baby is about the size of a rutabaga and moving constantly, positioning itself in all sorts of positions. But the baby primarily sits and stays in a breech position until later in the pregnancy. By now the baby may have found a precious thing—its thumb—and sucks on it frequently.

Mother—You are most likely feeling tired and you may find it's harder to get comfortable in bed. When riding in the car, wear your seatbelt under your tummy and across your chest to protect the baby. If you're driving, make sure you lift the steering wheel up and set the seat back or look into a Tummy Shield. Some women start to worry during this time of the pregnancy as they listen to other women's stories of pregnancy. Remember, those are their stories, not yours.

Flower—Mother-to-Be to Pick

This week, choose flowers that call to you and warm your heart. These flowers will put a smile on your face, as they are as beautiful as your pregnancy.

Crystal—Carnelian Agate

This crystal protects the wearer from allergens, which can invade your body at this time. Carnelian is about the feminine essence; it helps transform negative thinking into positive outcomes.

Color—Mother-to-Be to Pick

This week, wear colors that attract you: a white blouse or daring black T-shirt. If you feel like wearing something floral or striped, do it—even if it doesn't match with anything else you're wearing.

Chakra—All of Them

Fine-tuning the chakras is a fun exercise to do when you feel spiritually unbalanced. There are three ways to do this. One, have an orgasm; two, ride a roller coaster, which may not be suitable at this time; and three, sing the "Do-Re-Mi" song from *The Sound of Music* as loud and as many times as you can. Each musical note has a corresponding chakra they tune in to.

Sing it as many times as you wish throughout the rest of your pregnancy and say the affirmation below immediately after.

Music balances my spiritual growth and stability in life.

Essential Oil—Mother-to-Be to Pick

This week is about choosing life and what makes you feel good. Use an essential oil that you've connected to and that you feel understands your pregnant senses.

Bath

Pampering your skin throughout your pregnancy is comforting. Fill your tub, add three drops of blue food dye, a cup of Epsom salts, a few drops of lavender essential oil, and a tablespoon of baby oil.

Candle—White

White is simple, strengthening, and spiritual, not to mention calming. Seek spiritual guidance from your faith this week, the faith that comes from your gut. Know that it will be smooth sailing from now on.

Meditation

Make yourself comfortable in your quiet place. Relax while your candle emits peaceful energies while relaxing music plays in the background. Your flowers give a sense of beauty and peace. Hold your crystal in your hand. Take a few deep breaths to center yourself with universal forces. Visualize how much your baby has grown since your last meditation. See all the organs in their rightful place and functioning as they should, peacefully and whole-heartedly, while the baby's little heart beats steadily, gracefully, and most important, healthy.

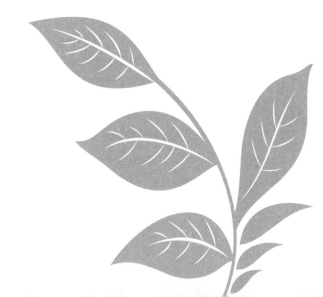

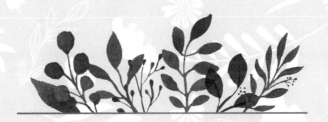

Week 26

I continue to bathe
in the light of sunshine.

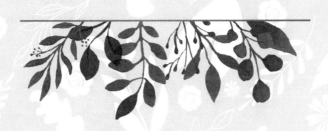

Baby—At this time, the baby has graduated to a head of lettuce. The baby's body is protected by a waxy surface called vernix. Vernix helps prevent the baby's skin from being irritated by urine, which the kidneys are now producing.

Mother—Your tummy is growing every day and there is nothing to stop it, so just go with the flow. Your breasts have started to produce colostrum, which is what the baby will ingest before your milk comes in. This is filled with nutrients and is very beneficial to the baby when first out of the womb.

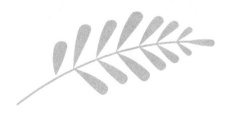

Flower—Pink Lilies

What a great time to bring these wonderful flowers back into your home. This time, use pink lilies, which represent love and partnership. These flowers will remind you to talk to your partner about your pregnancy so they don't feel left out.

Crystal—Moonstone

This crystal has the power to strengthen the mammary glands. It will induce milk that is rich in vitamins and minerals for your baby's growth and development out of the womb.

Color—Yellow

Yellow is a happy, receptive, and intuitive color. This week, wear yellow around your right wrist, or left wrist if you're left-handed. It could be a yellow band, ribbon, or even tape. Every time you see it, visualize yourself strengthening your intuitive connection with your child.

Chakra—Solar Plexus

The solar plexus can identify falseness in the people and the world you live in. This chakra can forewarn danger if you are receptive and listen. By using the below affirmation, you will encourage your baby's future life to be forewarned and for your child to listen to their instinct.

My child's intuition will be second to none.
It will guard his/her emotions throughout life.

Essential Oil—Sweet Orange

Use sweet orange in your oil burner or diffuser this week. Sweet orange brings peace and joy into the home, but best of all, it brings laughter. When you laugh, your baby is content and happy in its space.

Bath—Honey (Do Not Use Soap)

While you fill your bath, gently dab yourself all over with honey. Rub it gently into your skin, especially any dry patches or stretch marks that may have appeared. I know this is a messy exercise, but your skin will thank you. Once done, step into your bath and gently massage your skin until the honey is gone. Once out, pat yourself dry and feel the subtle softness of your skin, which is now nourished and loved.

Caution: Have someone help you in and out of the tub, as it could be slippery.

Candles—Blue and Purple

Burning these two candles together brings peace and harmony to the home. These will soothe any discomfort or tension in your relationships.

Meditation

This week's meditation is about nourishing your child. Go to your quiet place where your candles burn and your flowers are close. Play a peaceful classical piece of music, like Brahms's "Lullaby." Close your eyes and visualize your breasts growing and swollen with nothing but baby superfoods. Visualize your baby's thirst and hunger being satisfied with what nature has bestowed upon you, never allowing them to go hungry and always there to pacify with comfort and nourishment.

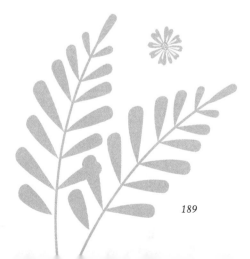

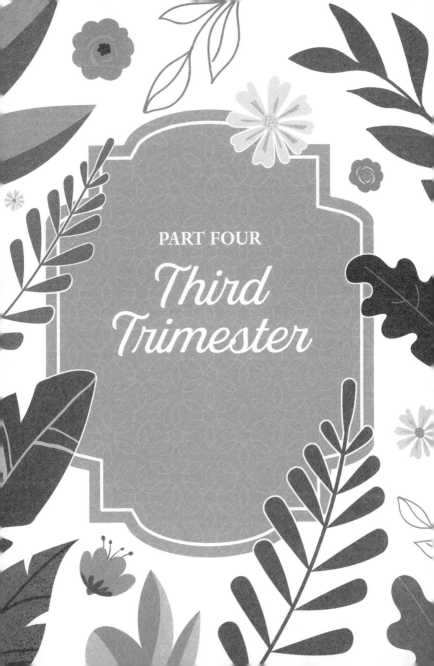

PART FOUR

Third Trimester

Tools Needed

Flowers

Freesias
Rosemary—Bunch
Gerberas—White
Carnations
Chrysanthemums—White
Calla Lily
Sunflowers
African Violets
Roses
Fennel—Bunch

Crystal

Aventurine
Clear Quartz
Fluorite
Rose Quartz
Obsidian
Amethyst
Hematite
Red Jasper
Garnet
Tiger Eye
Clear Calcite

Color

White
Violet
Red
Pink
Blue
Purple
Orange

Essential Oil

Ginger
Neroli (Orange Blossom)
Lavender
Lemon
Spearmint
Frankincense
Ylang-Ylang
Bergamot
Chamomile
Lime

Bath

Epsom Salts
Whole Milk
Wheat Germ Oil
Almond Oil
Oranges
Purple Food Dye

Candles

Purple
Pink
Yellow
Red
White
Blue
Green
Tea Lights
Silver

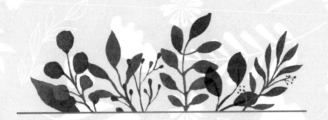

Week 27

I celebrate the beginning
of my third trimester.

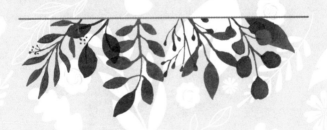

Baby—The baby is the size of a cauliflower. The baby fits snug in the uterus. The baby's eyelids are no longer fused together and are now open, making the baby more sensitive to the light passing through the abdominal wall.

Mother—Guess what? You've developed the *pregnancy waddle*. Think of it as cute. You are heavier and it's most likely getting harder for you to get around. Exercise or go for a walk—walking does wonders for our mental frame of mind, our weight, and, not to mention, our mobility throughout the pregnancy.

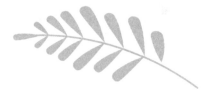

Flower—Freesias

Freesias express everything but negativity. Bring these beautiful aromatic flowers into your home this week. They will lift any solemn mood in the home and enhance the love that exists between you and your partner. They also bring health to your family, as well as the contentment of a very happy baby.

Crystal—Aventurine

In week 13 we used this crystal to communicate with the baby. Keep this crystal on hand for the rest of your pregnancy. It can be used as a mediator as it passes your energy to the baby.

Color—White

White is spiritual, positive, and the essence of innocence. Wear as much white as you can this week, and when you do, think of the little life you carry and wish it all that is positive in life.

Chakra—Third Eye

The third eye is linked to sight and intuition. The baby's eyes are open and already see light. This week is about giving your baby a chance to see things clearly in all of life's situations. By repeating the following affirmation at least three times a day this week, you can awaken intuition in your child's future.

The light my baby sees has love and endless possibilities.

Essential Oil–Frankincense

We used this wise oil in week 19 to reduce stress and tension, but it can also connect us with the spiritual world. When burning it on your oil burner or diffuser, this oil purifies all that is good and beautiful. It protects the things you love while giving your pregnancy a sense of knowing that everything is going to be all right.

Bath

Once again, it's time for a relaxing massage in the bath. It will help with your sleeping patterns while smoothing your tangled muscles and thoughts for you to effectively get some sleep.

Candle–Purple and Pink

These colors together strengthen the faith within and the ability to see the goodness in people even in their worst moments. These candles will aid your child to see the light beyond what we see without any emotional shutters.

Meditation

Go to your meditation space and listen to a song from your playlist, preferably something delicate and moving. Look at your candles burning and the flowers that are so happy to be in your home. Smell the essence of your essential oil and close your eyes. Take a few deep breaths and relax.

Visualize your baby's eyes and what they now see and what they will see in their future. Visualize acute vision, not only physically but spiritually. Visualize your child seeing the world in a positive light, filtering the best and worst of people without judgement.

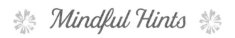
Weight Gain

At this point in your pregnancy, you've noticed the weight gain. How can you not with all those weigh-ins at your prenatal visits like a jockey before a race? Your medical provider should tell you if you're on track with your weight gain or if you're over or under. If you're on track, walk out with a smile on your face because everything is as it should be.

I find a lot of women complain about their weight and want it gone within a few days after giving birth. If it took you forty weeks to gain the weight, it may take you just as long to lose it all, to fit into those skinny jeans again, and to get back to pre-pregnancy weight.

Pregnancy and weight gain go hand-in-hand—it's just the way it is. Going on a diet while pregnant is not advisable. The smart thing to do is maintain a healthy, well-balanced diet full of the good things your baby needs for its growth and development. When you do, you'll provide the baby with the best nutrients you can possibly give.

When you gain weight, it's a due process. Who cares? This is the first time in your life when you can gain weight and have an excuse for it! But it doesn't mean you're eating for two. You're eating for one and nourishing the other. This doesn't give you carte blanche to eat all those yummy chocolates. Well, maybe a little, but don't overdo something that you know is not good for you while pregnant or thereafter.

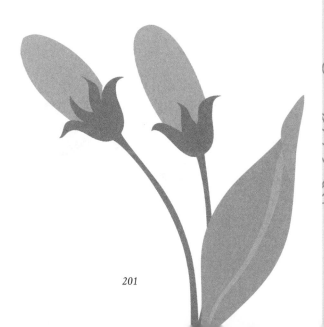

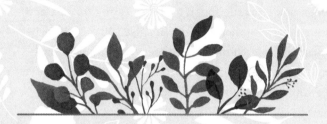

Week 28

Love resides inside my womb.

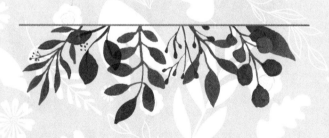

Baby—The baby has graduated to the size of a large eggplant. The lungs continue to develop. Brain-waves increase while millions of new brain cells form. The cerebral cortex can now send electrical impulses through the baby's body.

Mom—Pregnancy hormones increase the flow of blood to the breasts, causing tissue changes and making the veins very prominent. Backaches could be an issue at this time. Your work may begin to exhaust you and you may start to wonder if you should start your maternity leave sooner rather than later.

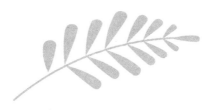

Flower—Bunch of Rosemary (Herb)

This week calls for a bunch of fresh rosemary again. Take out all the leaves and put them in a red silk drawstring bag. Take it to work or anywhere you need to focus. Inhale the fragrance. You're not only enhancing your concentration, but enhancing the baby's brain activities as well.

Crystal—Clear Quartz

This crystal is an eraser of the things we fear. If you have something you wish to erase, like fear of the ocean or spiders, this is the crystal to have. By letting go of fear, you will not pass your fear into your child's world.

Color—Violet

Violet is an amazing color that strengthens the way we walk and live in life. Use a violet-colored pencil and draw what you think your baby's brain and your brain look like. Then draw a rope to link them together. This exercise is to keep you in tune with your child in the future. Always keep this drawing in a special place.

Chakra—Crown

This week is all about the baby's brain as it develops its own characteristics and infinite possibilities. As the baby's chakras come to life, the affirmation below can help connect them to Universal wisdom.

My baby's brain is immeasurable, just like the Universe.

Essential Oil—Mother-to-Be to Pick

This week, pick an essential oil that you've previously enjoyed and use it for the same reason it was used in past weeks. It may relate to something you need this week.

Bath

Use Epsom salts this week to alleviate the discomfort of sore muscles. Add a half-cup of wheat germ oil or almond oil to soothe and nourish your skin from dryness.

Caution: Have someone help you in and out of the tub, as it could be slippery.

Candle—Yellow

Whenever you see the flame of this very perceptive candle, visualize your future child studying and making it a fun experience. See your child applying themselves to math, science, or whatever they wish to excel in.

Meditation

Take a few deep breaths while you relax in your quiet place. Enjoy the flicker of the candle's flame and smell your chosen essential oil. Hold the clear quartz crystal in one hand and the drawstring bag containing rosemary in the other. Play a meaningful song in the background.

Visualize your child at this time in your pregnancy. See your baby's brain engulfed by electrical charges connecting each sensor to its fullest potential. See your child's brain work and function to enhance its potential. Visualize your child's mind flourishing in art, intelligence, empathy, common sense, compassion, and, most important, the ability to feel love and to be loved.

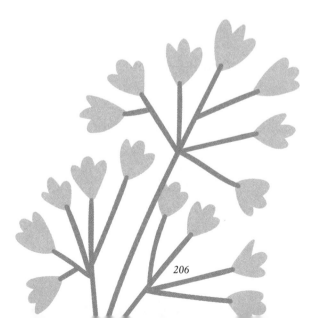

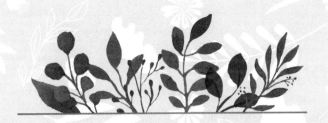

Week 29

My pregnancy is health incarnate.

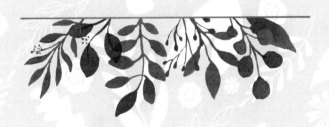

Baby—The baby is now a little more than three pounds and about the size of an acorn squash. The baby is practicing breathing movements as it swallows amniotic fluid. The nervous system is more complex and the baby is filling out more with muscle and fat. The baby's weight will double between now and birth.

Mother—Heartburn and constipation keep making an entrance. Your ribs make way for the baby and, in turn, make your lungs work harder. You may be tired and less motivated to do things. It's now time to start with your pelvic floor exercises to improve your bladder control, and strengthen your pelvic muscles for a better recovery after childbirth.

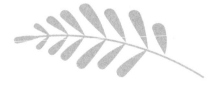

Flower—White Gerberas

In week 13 we used gerberas to celebrate entering the second trimester. This week, bring white gerberas into your home to ground you. They will also give you the stability needed to navigate the chaos of everyday life to ensure things are resolved with a positive outcome.

Crystal—Fluorite

As you did in week 18, keep this crystal by your bedside or under your pillow. It aids with the health and development of the baby's bone and gum structure and it helps you with the aches of bone and muscle discomfort at this stage of your pregnancy.

Color—Red

Wear red this week, even if it's a band around your hair or lace around your wrist. It will give you an extra oomph of energy whenever you look at it.

Chakra—Root

Pregnancy is an emotional roller coaster. The ups and downs you go through affect all chakras and can make them overactive or underactive. When the root chakra is balanced, the other chakras will be as well.

Say the following affirmation as often as you need to ensure your root chakra and all other chakras stay balanced.

My emotions are the strings of a musical instrument and are in tune with one another.

Essential Oil—Ginger

Once again, use ginger essential oil, the multitasker. It can soothe, excite, energize, and enhance anything you want or need. If finances are low, bring the ginger essence into your home to invigorate them.

Caution: This essential oil is strong and spicy, so start with one drop at a time.

Bath—Swimming

You need buoyancy right now, so go for a swim. Don't go to a surf beach, but rather somewhere calm so you can float and alleviate the pressure on your back. A heated pool is best to relax your muscles and emotions.

Candles—Red

Get a red candle and light it while thinking of the energy you need. It will give you the same extra bounce in your step that wearing red does.

Spiritual Boost

Take your partner for a nature walk. Hold hands and talk about the baby while surrounded by the things in nature that make you breathe peace and calm. Enjoy your time alone together because if this is your first baby, there will soon be three of you.

If you already have kids, go on a family outing. Discuss with your other child or children what they are best at and give that child the responsibility to teach those qualities to the new baby when the time comes.

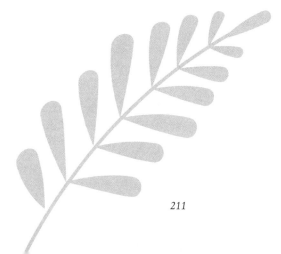

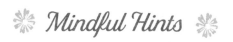

❄ *Mindful Hints* ❄

Troubled Sleep

Getting comfortable in bed is a major issue at this time and the lack of sleep can make you feel tired, irritable, and unproductive. The back-and-forth trips to the bathroom can be annoying, which add to the nightly fray. When you eventually get some sleep, your dreams can be so vivid that you'll remember them for the rest of your life.

All your restlessness to seek comfort and sleep is attributed to the growth of the baby, who is also trying to find comfort in their own space. As the baby grows, they start to press and kick important organs like the kidneys, liver, and bladder, which can cause discomfort.

To avoid some of those discomforts, there are things you can try to help get you through these non-sleep times:

- Take a lavender bath with Epsom salts before bedtime.
- Drink a cup of chamomile tea to settle your mind and muscles.
- Sleep on your left side to avoid organs like the liver.

- Cut out caffeine.
- Avoid rigorous exercise before bed.
- Stay away from social media or any computer/phone/tablet screens before bed.
- Eat smaller meals at night.
- If you can't sleep, get up, read a book (not on a tablet), and drink a cup of decaf herbal tea or a glass of warm milk with honey or dash of nutmeg until you feel relaxed enough to go back to bed.
- Hold an amethyst crystal in your hand or to your chest to help you find sleep.
- Rub drops of lavender on your pillow.
- Get your partner to rub your shoulders or give you a foot rub.
- If your lack of sleep is due to pregnancy concerns, talk to your medical provider to ease your worries.
- Take a pregnancy yoga class for relaxation techniques.
- If you can, take a nap during the day to catch up on sleep.
- Talk to your baby to settle any discomfort the baby may have due to your restlessness.

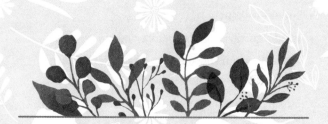

Week 30

I am here in the now
and emotionally minded
with my loved ones.

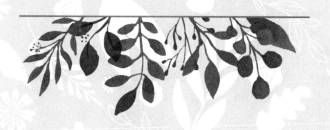

Baby—The baby is growing and getting bigger every day. It's about the size of a cabbage right now. The baby is tucked in nicely and sitting on its bottom. Even if it's started to get a little cramped in its space, the baby is still flexible enough to move around. The baby has also started acquiring sleeping patterns, hopefully mirrored to yours!

Mother—Even though labor is in approximately ten weeks, your uterus is already starting to prepare for the event, both physically and emotionally. Your bathroom visits are more frequent, and your focus may be scattered somewhere in baby la-la land, so talk to your partner to keep you grounded and focused.

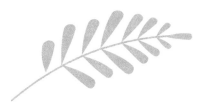

Flower—Carnations

Buy a bunch of multicolored carnations for your home. These resilient little buds will help you keep your emotions in check for the week.

Crystal—Rose Quartz

While pregnant, we may get so caught up within our own thoughts that we forget what's important and that not everyone is pregnant. You may have even neglected your family emotionally. This crystal will help you find the resources to spread yourself around to those you love and who love you. Rub it on your stomach and pass along the love you feel for your baby.

Color—Pink

Pink will help you to stay cool and collected, communicate with your loved ones, and banish resentful feelings that may hover around you at this time. Don't attribute all your feelings to hormones. Be sure to think before you act, and you'll stay in the realm of the wise.

Chakra—Solar Plexus

This chakra is intuitive and understands turmoil. This chakra's mantra is *the fire within each one of us*. It activates and increases our energy and emotional intuitiveness on life so you can foresee your baby's needs.

Say the following to stay focused on your intuitive nature.

I listen and feel the rhythm of life
within me and that of my baby.

Essential Oil—Neroli (Orange Blossom)

This happy oil brings alertness and fun to the home. It gives the baby the warm fuzzies in your womb. When you create happiness, the baby will enjoy the endorphins just as much as you do.

Bath

Place the peels of three oranges into the tub while it fills. Add a few drops of lavender essential oil, four drops of purple food dye, and a cup of Epsom salts. Sink into this bath and enjoy the reflective peacefulness it brings.

Candle—White

Write your due date on a white tapered candle. Light the candle and visualize the month and season the baby will be born in. Make sure the candle lasts for the seven days of week 30. Every day when you light the candle, you'll reinforce the due date and embed this stage of your pregnancy with love, trust, and light.

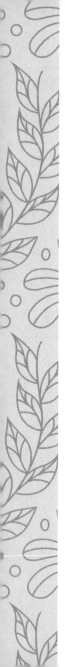

Spiritual Boost

Read your journal up until this point of your pregnancy. Add anything you've forgotten, pictures you've taken, and special mementos such as visits to your care provider, the baby's weight, and your weight. Write about significant moments of your pregnancy thus far or add a weekly affirmation to your journey to reflect on later in life or your next pregnancy.

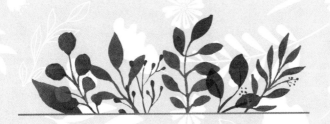

Week 31

My tummy is a sign that my baby
is developing and growing
strong and healthy.

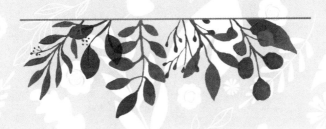

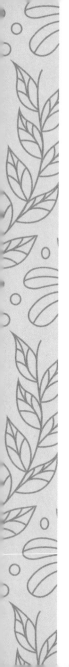

Baby—Well, now the baby is approximately the size of a spaghetti squash and exercises their limbs regularly. Movements become stronger and they may startle you at times. Playing music for the baby will help connect the synapses of the baby's brain.

Mother—Your prenatal appointments will increase as you get ready for your delivery day. Keep a list of the baby's movements in your journal. It gives you and your care provider an idea of what the baby is doing.

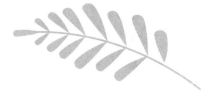

Flower—Baby's Choice

Go to a florist or a supermarket's flower section. Stand in front of all the flowers. Look at them and pat your tummy and silently ask your baby, "Which ones?" Close your eyes and let your baby guide you to the essence it needs. When you open your eyes, there will be one that beckons you above the others. Take those ones home and display them while visualizing faith in your future parenting skills.

Crystal—Obsidian

This crystal is good at dispelling negativity, should you have any as your due date gets closer. It also aids with skin conditions such as dryness or acne and alleviates sinusitis, which can manifest through pregnancy.

Color—Mother-to-Be to Pick

This week, wear something nice from your maternity wardrobe. Go to your hairdresser and have your hair done. Smile each morning when you walk out the door and know that the energy a pregnant woman exudes is filled with love and life.

Chakra—Sacral

Your sacral chakra and uterus are working extra hard to hold life. This week, affirm the hard work they're both doing in the development of your baby, which is crucial to your pregnancy.

I thank my uterus for all its hard work and my sacral chakra for helping me through this wonderful experience.

Essential Oil—Lavender

Bring lavender into your home once again to settle the baby and bring peace to their restless little body as they look to get comfortable.

Bath

As you progress into your pregnancy, make sure someone is home when you take a bath. They will be able to help you get in and out, making sure you don't slip and fall.

This week, experiment with your bath. Don't be shy. Put in anything that comes to mind. You may even put in all the crystals you've used thus far, or just the ones that say, "Yep, I'll go for a swim."

Caution: Put the crystal(s) in after you get into the bath and take them out before you get out.

Family Candle Meditation

This week, ask your partner to meditate with you for a few minutes. If you have any other children who are old enough to sit still for a few minutes, have them join in. Light a white candle for each person and one for the baby. Sit where you are most comfortable and hold hands. Have your essential oil fill the room and use your flowers as a focal point.

Ask everyone to close their eyes and guide them through this meditation as you describe the essence of the baby using your senses. Tell them how it feels to have a life growing within you. Tell them what you think the baby thinks about them, which will certainly amuse your little ones.

Have fun with this family meditation and take it wherever you want it to take you.

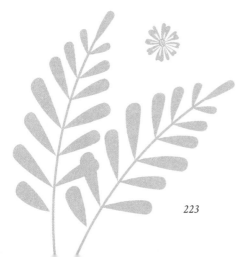

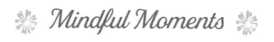# *Mindful Moments*

Baby Shower

A baby shower is when family and friends get together to shower you with "baby happiness." Baby showers celebrate the new life coming into this plane of existence and rejoice in the momentous occasion that is to come. This is a precious moment in your life, so take lots of pictures to put in your journal. You can look back on and smile at those precious moments later in life.

You and your bundle are the center of attention of this joyous occasion, surrounded by loved ones who want to share in your wonderful experience. And the good thing about your baby shower is that you just need to show up, so you can let a family member or friend take over the task of planning it.

Family or friends often go in on a gift you need, like a stroller or something similar. The rest of your guests may bring clothes, blankets, and toiletries for your baby—they may even supply you with newborn diapers for the first week. If you're trying to lessen the environmental impact of the diapers you use, be sure to alert people that you plan to use cloth diapers so they will purchase the correct gift.

Enjoy the food and cupcakes, which are often decorated in traditional blue or pink. There are also games to play and they can be a lot of fun. There may be baby name-guessing games, a belly-painting session, or you may get a belly casting kit or session. Whatever you receive, enjoy it and be thankful for this magical experience.

Don't forget to bring the hostess or hostesses flowers or another gift for making it all happen. Thank them for their efforts and let them know how much it means to you. The flowers will convey your appreciation and they'll love receiving them.

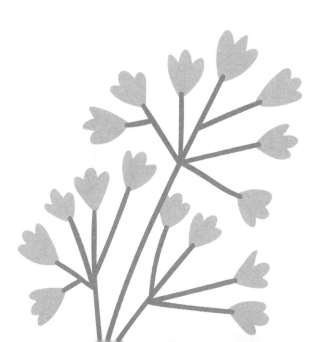

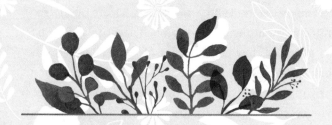

Week 32

My baby feels my touch
and smiles at the comfort it brings.

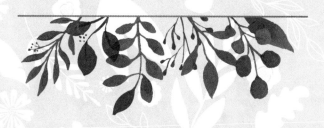

Baby—Baby is around the size of a papaya and is active touching their face and pulling on their umbilical cord. The baby has become a little contortionist because of the flexibility of their limbs. The skin is a little more opaque and is not as see-through as it was previously. They could already be in the engaged position, which is bottom-up, ready for birth.

Mother—Your heart rate may increase and at times you may feel it flutter. Your belly button may protrude, but it usually goes back to normal after birth. It seems like your body is no longer your own. The skin around your midsection keeps stretching. Make sure you get as much fiber as you can to stay regular. And you may find yourself a little clumsy, so know your limitations.

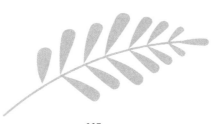

Flower—White Chrysanthemums

We used these flowers in week 10 to convey trust to your child and to let them know you'll always be there for them. These flowers are also excellent for calming your anxious heart and mind for what's ahead.

Crystal—Amethyst

Right about now you may need a little peace and self-assurance. An amethyst can give you that. It will keep you calm, not only emotionally, but also physically from all pregnancy ailments.

Color—Purple

Purple will bounce spirituality back into your life. This is the color of the masters and souls who have visited our plane of existence over many lifetimes. Every time you wear purple this week, you'll further connect with your child on a spiritual level.

Chakra—Crown

The crown chakra is our connection to all that is within us and around us.

This week, make that connection with your baby and feel enlightened that you're not only linked physically, but also spiritually. The below affirmation confirms the commitment of your spiritual bond.

My baby and I share a spiritual bond that binds us together.

Essential Oil—Lemon

In week 10 we used lemon to aid nausea, but lemon's energy is also get-up-and-go. This oil will help get rid of the pregnancy sloth feeling you may experience and get you up and about to finish unfinished tasks while brightening your day with its freshness.

Massage

This week, ask your partner to give you a relaxing massage that's tender and loving. Make sure they rub your feet and the back of your calves using pregnancy-friendly carrier oils such as almond oil.

Candle—Purple and Blue

The combination of these two candles brings nothing but protective energies to the home. It shifts your thoughts from worry to confidence.

Spiritual Boost

Now that you've had your baby shower, cross off the things you no longer need to purchase due to the gifts you and your baby were given. Making sure you have everything on this list can be a fun activity, but it can be an expensive undertaking, especially for bigger items like cribs. If this isn't your first pregnancy, you may still have things from your first child. If you do, clean them and spruce them up for the new baby if they're a bit weathered. If this is your first pregnancy, do your homework before you get a car seat or crib. See which brand is the safest and most economical. Remember, they will grow out of clothes and furniture like strollers and high chairs. As far as clothes go, all they need are a few outfits and a Sunday best.

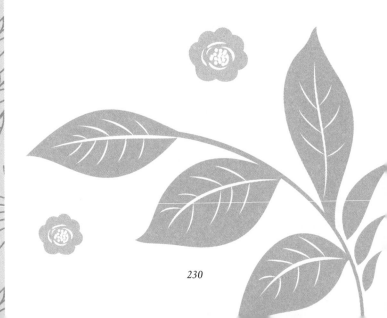

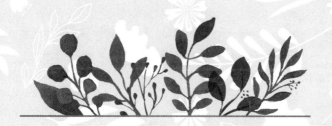

Week 33

I let my skin stretch
to accommodate my baby.

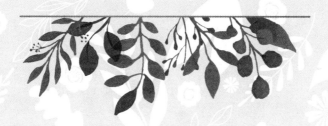

Baby—The baby resembles a small baby doll at this time. There will not be large changes from now on, only development. The kidneys and lungs could function out of the womb around this time and amniotic fluid is at maximum capacity.

Mother—The baby presses on your bladder and accidents could happen. You may feel your body is no longer yours. The skin around your midsection keeps stretching and it gets drier.

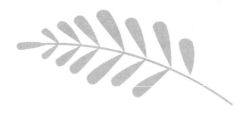

Flower—White Calla Lily

Displaying calla lilies in your home will make you more aware of the things you want to do and the reasons why you want to do them, like getting the baby's room ready and listening to your gut feeling.

Crystal—Hematite

This is a great crystal for any type of insecurities you may feel. It also helps you reach your goals before you go into labor. Just have it at arm's reach from now on, as you never know when you're going to need it.

Color—Blue

Blue is a great color to use to stay calm and to find sleep. It's time to trade your purple pajamas for a blue pair to keep you and the baby calm and to get restful sleep.

Chakra / Shower

It's time to sing the "Do-Re-Mi" song from *The Sound of Music* again. This time, sing it while in the shower. Let the water element wash away the emotions of the day while you sing. Right after your shower, say the affirmation below. As you do, you nourish all seven life points of your body with emotional food and well-being.

For my unborn child, I nourish the life centers of my body with positive emotional thoughts and actions.

Essential Oil—Spearmint

We used this oil in week 9 to alleviate morning sickness, but it also keeps the home happy and blissful when burned in your oil burner or diffuser.

Candle—Green

Green is the color of growth and understanding. It helps to heal old emotional wounds and create happy new ones. As the candle burns, it will help you to be the mother you always wanted to be and heal your heart from past hurts and sorrows.

Meditation

Head to your meditation space. See the light of your green candle and the beauty of the calla lilies while you let the scent of the oil fill you with peace and love. Make sure you're comfortable while you hold the hematite crystal, taking deep, controlled breaths. Close your eyes and see your pregnancy thus far—the ups and downs with the aches and all. Then visualize the joy the life inside you is feeling because you've given your baby understanding and a warm, loving space.

Now, tune in to your baby's physical needs and make sure they are all being met. Visualize each pink organ soaking up the nutrients and emotional stability you've given them with your love and the positive outlook you bring to your pregnancy.

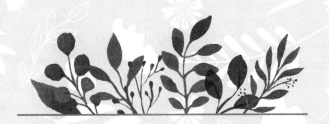

Week 34

Even if I now waddle,
I waddle in style.

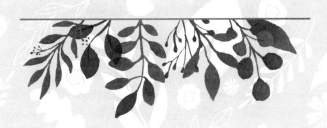

Baby—The baby is about the size of a pineapple and looks more in proportion to its body and is nicely plump. The bones continue to harden. The pupils of the eyes dilate when exposed to light through the womb.

Mother—You may have started to experience hot flashes and may opt to wear cooler clothing, even in winter. The baby's movements are stronger and more frequent. Exfoliate your tummy to get rid of dry skin. You will still be suffering through all the delights of pregnancy like a sore back and acid reflux.

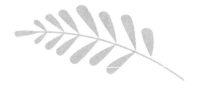

Flowers—Sunflowers

These yellow pieces of sunlight bring happiness to the home, intuition to those who display them, and purity of the heart to the soul. This week, dedicate these flowers to your baby with open affection and unconditional love.

Crystal—Red Jasper

We used red jasper in week 12 to strengthen your mind from baby brain syndrome. Now is the time to bring back this crystal until the end of your pregnancy to activate all dormant brain cells and the baby's brain cells.

Color—Mother-to-Be to Pick

Choose a color for the baby's room if you haven't already. Don't feel foolish if you want to consult your baby. Bring some large pieces of colored cardboard into the room to see how the baby reacts to each in the sunlight. Keep your colors warm and not neon-bright. You want the baby to feel comforted, not alarmed by a bright red, purple, or even green. Go softer; pastel colors are wonderful for a baby's room.

Chakra

At this time the baby has all its chakras. The third eye and the crown chakras will develop more after birth, but even now the baby is in tune with emotions. It may be on a smaller scale, but the emotions are present. You know when the baby is uncomfortable or unsettled by the force of the kicks they give you. So yes, emotions are there and every time you feel these discomforts, say the affirmation below to affirm these beliefs to the baby.

I feel what you feel and am in tune with your comforts and your discomforts.

Essential Oil—Frankincense

Use frankincense essential oil this week to balance the baby's little chakras, to seek harmony within the baby's spiritual center, and to feel connected to the world that it will be born into.

Bath—Swimming

Again, go for a swim or float in a heated pool. The water will help take pressure off your entire pregnant body, but most important, your back. Float as much as you can and enjoy the feeling.

Candles—Red and Green

Together these two candles are a force to be reckoned with. Red signifies strength and courage and green signifies growth and healing. When these colors are used together it gives you that extra oomph to get the things done that you haven't tackled yet or finish the ones you've started previously.

Spiritual Boost

Do something fun outdoors that you'll enjoy. You may want to garden or re-pot some indoor plants. You might go to a local market or take a romantic trip with your partner. Prepare a dinner you've been dying to attempt or bake something yummy. Or just sloth for the day— slothing around is always good for the soul. But whatever you do, enjoy it to the fullest. You can even go on a babymoon around this time to enjoy time together before the big day!

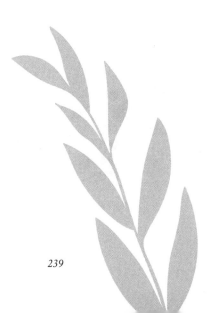

Week 35

I give and receive love freely
at this stage of my pregnancy.

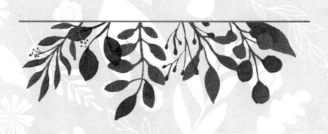

Baby—On the fruit-and-vegetable scale, your baby may be the size of a butternut squash or pumpkin right now. The baby could be in the engaged position in preparation for the exit in a few weeks' time. The baby is not doing much except gaining weight and growing happily.

Mother—You have probably started the countdown. You could be more emotional. If the baby is in the engaged position, it released pressure on your diaphragm and makes it easier to breathe. The baby could be putting more pressure on your bladder, which means more bathroom breaks and sleep-ins are off the table.

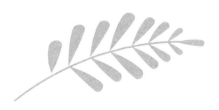

Flower—African Violets

Bring home a pot of these calming, purple flowers to help soothe the next couple of weeks and to bring peace of mind and protect you from self-inflicted thoughts.

Crystal—Amethyst and Garnet

Together these two crystals bring peace, harmony, and good health when carried or worn. They bring positive thought patterns and help free your mind from worrisome health issues related to your pregnancy.

Color—Purple

Reaching a higher sense of consciousness to communicate with the baby is reassuring while pregnant, not only for you, but for the baby as well. Wear purple this week to give you a spiritual sense of belonging in a cosmic balance with the baby.

Chakra—Root

Once again, emotions come out to play and could affect the normalcy of things. Happiness and sadness might present themselves without warning and can be overwhelming. It could be that your root chakra is unbalanced and needs reassurance, which is normal during this time of pregnancy. The affirmation below will stabilize your emotional center.

I heal my emotions by staying healthy, grounded,
and balanced with the oneness of who I am
and who I am meant to be to myself and my baby.

Essential Oil—Ylang-Ylang

In week 12 you used this oil to stay in focus, be grateful, and to express love. It's a good idea to express gratitude that at 35 weeks, you are happy, healthy, and well, and to bring resolution to any health or emotional problems you have been dealing with.

Bath

It could be getting harder to get in and out of the tub right about now. Make sure there is always someone there to help you when you take a bath.

This week, relax your muscles with Epsom salts. Add a few drops of lavender and ylang-ylang to the bath. These two oils will calm your emotions and balance your anxious heart when you breathe in their loving, positive energies. These energies settle the baby, readying them for the birth.

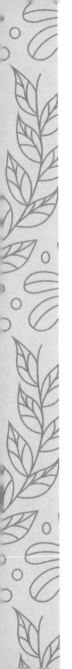

Candle Meditation

Light twelve tea light candles around your meditation space. Turn all the lights down or off and snuggle into a comfortable position on your couch, floor, or yoga mat. Don't forget to play your favorite relaxing music. Breathe in the scent of your essential oil. Notice the African violets in the background bringing peace and harmony to you and your baby.

Take a few deep breaths and tune in to your baby and what they're doing at this time of your pregnancy. Visualize the baby's heart beating happily while blood flows throughout their little body. Visualize the baby's major organs functioning, circulating clean and untarnished positive energy now and throughout their life.

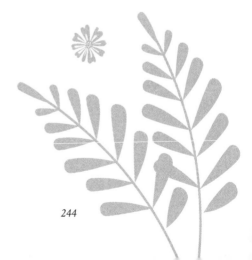

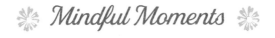

Mindful Moments

Nesting

From now until the end of the pregnancy, women typically experience what's called "nesting." Nesting is an instinct that cannot be stopped. It occurs when every part of your mind and body wants to get ready for this baby, no matter the time of day. You might feel like everything must be perfect, clean, and sparkling, as if important visitors are coming.

If you haven't already, now is a good time to start getting the baby's room ready, which may feel like it needed to be done yesterday. You may want to clean the entire house. Just remember you can't do it at two in the morning or you'll wake the entire household, even if you are fired up to do it.

First, make a list of the things you want to accomplish and review it with your partner. Tick things off when they're finished. This paranormal energy (as I call it) after feeling sluggish for so long is like an emotional high. Don't do silly things like stepping on a ladder or using paints, which can give off fumes that may be bad for you and the baby. You may feel energized, but you're still pregnant, so take care. But most of all, enjoy the preparation because you have a beautiful, permanent tenant on the way.

Week 36

Life cannot get any better than I feel.

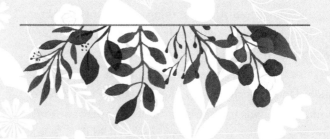

Baby—The baby is almost full-term and is around the size of a honeydew melon. The lungs are up and running, and so are all the other major organs. The average weight for this week is around 5.5 pounds. Remember, the baby can hear your voice, so keep talking to your child. They won't have a clue what you're saying, but the tone of your voice matters.

Mother—You may have started your maternity leave. You may soon experience sporadic Braxton-Hicks contractions. Besides the lack of sleep and aches and pains of pregnancy, you may experience short bursts of nesting energy. You may enjoy the boost of energy, which has likely been absent.

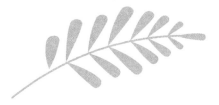

Flower—Roses

Pick a colorful bunch of roses for the home this week. They bring peace to the home and to you and the baby. The different colors embrace new beginnings for you and your family.

Crystal—Tiger Eye

This crystal will bring confidence, courage, and good luck while being very protective. It also strengthens the womb and the elasticity that's needed, so keep it close by or under your pillow.

Color—Orange

Wear orange around your stomach area these upcoming weeks. If you don't have a pair of orange underwear, skirt, or pants, get an orange ribbon and wrap it around your tummy to strengthen the cervix for its finest upcoming moments.

Chakra—Sacral

As your pregnancy nears the end, the sacral chakra could still be making you feel sensitive and emotional, which is normal. You might feel like crying at the drop of a hat. By saying the below affirmation, you'll find the strength to cope with this week's challenges.

I am in control and my life force shines within me.

Essential Oil—Bergamot

This essential oil brings light and sunshine to your home. Burn it on your oil burner or diffuser to bring harmony and love to cherish your baby, even if the baby makes your last few weeks uncomfortable.

Shower

In a one-liter container, blend a cup of whole milk, two drops of lavender, and two drops of chamomile and top off the container with warm water. Turn your shower to your preferred temperature. Use your washcloth to anoint your body with this milky-scented lotion. As you do, feel peace and know the baby enjoys the scent while your dry skin loves the moisture.

Caution: Make sure you have a non-slip mat in the shower and someone to help you out.

Candle—White and Yellow

These colored candles bring harmony and peace to the home when burned together. They can enhance the baby's brain activities to process endorphins.

Spiritual Boost

Even though you're in your last weeks, there is always time for a walk or whatever activity keeps you active and fit. It's a good idea to not do much on your own, so take a buddy. There are several people who would love to pamper and keep you company. If you've been doing yoga, concentrate on your breathing. It will help with labor.

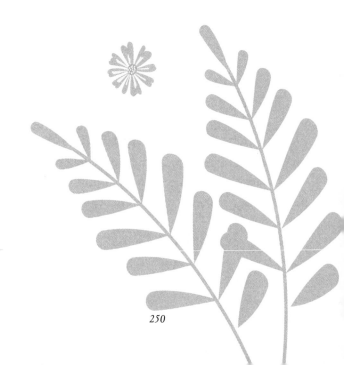

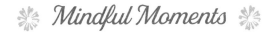

Mindful Moments

Naming the Baby

Naming your child is not an easy task and carries a lot of responsibility. Take your time choosing a name until you know it's the right one for your child. After all, they will carry it throughout their lifetime.

Some people wait until they see the baby before they choose a name. Others know before they get pregnant. Some choose names for their strength and courageous representation that will hearten their child's existence. You might choose a family name.

If you don't know the gender of the baby, make a list of both the boy and girl names you like. Once you have a substantial list, start culling names. Don't let your personal opinions dictate the name of your child, like if someone you don't like or a famous personality that irritates you has the name you're considering.

Names can sometimes be a fad that pass through our life like hurricane season. Some don't cause damage while others tear the earth apart. Some names are timeless, like Charles, Edward, Mary, or Lily. A lot of new parents consider similar names for their simplicity and uncomplicated meaning.

It's time to narrow down your list to three boys' names and three girls' names. Think the names over and try saying the names out loud to your partner. Brainstorm the nicknames your child may have. For example, see if you like people changing the name Nicholas to Nick, Nico, or Nicki or the name Samantha to Sam, Sammy, or Simi. Many names have nicknames, including the endearing ones you give your child according to their personality. Apply the same logic to middle names that sometimes become first names as your child ages.

So do your homework, light a white candle for inspiration and guidance, and hold a rose quartz crystal throughout the elimination process to guide you to the name your child will love and treasure.

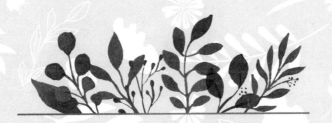

Week 37

My baby and I have
started the countdown.

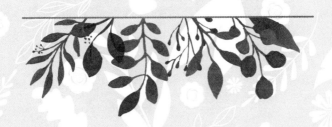

Baby—The baby fruit-and-vegetable guide tells us the baby is about the size of a winter melon. Currently, extra space within the womb is limited, which makes the baby go into a more fetal position.

Mother—Your movements may be slow and difficult, and even maintaining balance could be a challenge. Milk ducts have created a milk delivery system for your baby. Mood swings can happen, so think before you act so you don't undo all the hard work you've done so far.

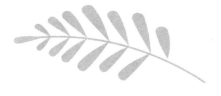

Flower—Bunch of Fennel (Herb)

Bring a fresh bunch of fennel home and display it as if it were flowers. This herb will aid in purifying the blood that flows through your body and in turn purify the baby. It is also a healing conduit to unknown illnesses, aches, and pains.

Crystal—Clear Calcite

From now until the end of your pregnancy, carry a piece of clear calcite with you. It will help strengthen your bones and teeth. It can also help with hypertension.

Color—White

This color has no agenda. White is pure and engenders trust. By wearing white this week, it will awaken spiritual awareness and help you to find comfort in knowing that all is as it should be and will be.

Chakra—Crown

It's time to bring faith to the table. It could be the faith of spiritual awareness, faith in the self, or faith in the Universe. Whichever faith you believe in, trust, or worship, this is the faith that motivates this chakra. The affirmation below will enlighten your faith.

My baby is at peace,
enlightened, and connected to the Divine.

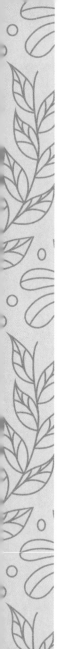

Essential Oil—Lime

This essential oil revitalizes the mind, uplifts your mood, and enhances physical energy, which you and the baby may need in the upcoming weeks as you ready for labor.

Bath—Foot Spa

You're ready for another foot spa and a much-needed pedicure about this time. It's not easy painting your toenails when you can't even bend down in a graceful manner. Let someone massage those tired, sore feet. Pick a color for your toenails that makes you happy and that revitalizes you.

Candles—Silver

This candle's color is associated with spirituality and fertility. This color is the fertility of life and connects to Mother Nature and its wonders. It's just the connection needed to stay grounded as you ready yourself and your baby for birth and life thereafter.

Birthing Classes and Focal Point

By this time, you've finished your birthing classes. These classes introduce you to labor and how to cope with the birthing ritual, including breathing exercises and how to remain focused. If you haven't taken one already, it's not too late to enroll in a class, as they're definitely worth it.

You may be thinking about what to use as your primary focal point throughout the labor process. This could be anything you can relate to that keeps you focused during the most stressful parts of childbirth. This focal point will be your mantra, your savior, and your belief to know everything will be all right. Whatever you choose, hold it in your hands and give it a purpose. If it's a photo, hold it to your heart and breath in the memories that will hold you together. If it's something that was your mother's or a special gift, hold it in your hands while visualizing a stress-free childbirth. Picture it soothing the worries of labor and keeping you focused throughout the birthing experience.

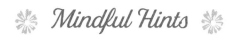

Mindful Hints

Hospital and Home Readiness

Hospital

It's a good idea to have your bag ready if you're going to have a hospital delivery instead of a home birth. The last thing you need to do is look for your favorite pair of slippers in the middle of a contraction, so start packing. From this point on, labor can manifest at any time. There are lists of what to take to the hospital that you can download from the internet, or better yet, make your own.

Pack a light bag with only the essentials and don't forget your maternity bra if you're not already wearing it. If there are no complications, you could be back home within twenty-four hours, but should you have a C-section, you could be there for three or more days. If you forget something, don't worry. A friend or family member can get it for you. Even your partner can do it if they're not staying overnight with you.

You've likely already taken the obligatory maternity tour at the hospital. This is a great exercise to complete so you know where everything is and what to expect when labor begins. When you arrive at the hospital for childbirth, one of the first things they will ask you is when was your last contraction and how far apart they are. So once they begin, take note of their frequency on a piece of paper or on your smartphone. Be ready for other questions from the hospital staff, such as who your OB/GYN is and what medical insurance you have. Make sure all your paperwork is up-to-date and your insurance coverage is at the ready.

Well-wishers sometimes show up unexpectedly at the hospital. It may make you uncomfortable to have visitors while you're not at your best or tired from an exhausting labor. Remember, you make the rules as to who or when to see friends and family. This is something you can discuss with them prior to labor. You may want just you and your partner in the delivery room. Don't feel guilty about your decisions. Your family will just have to understand and respect your wishes. But make sure they're known before you end up in the hospital battling through a room of uninvited people à la *My Big Fat Greek Wedding*.

Home

Home delivery is totally different. You don't have to pack a bag, but you do need to get yourself ready just as you would if you were going to the hospital. First, create a space. Call it your sacred birthing space, a space that can be cleaned thoroughly after the birth. Once this is done, this space is given a purpose and creates the desired spiritual atmosphere.

Gather sheets and towels; make sure they're clean and ready for use. Look into renting a birthing tub. Ask your midwife or doula for help in this matter. They will guide you as to what is best. After all, they've done this many times and know what's best for the birth.

Make sure you have plan B ready should it arise. Have the phone number for your local hospital somewhere everyone can see. Also have your purse, insurance information, and emergency transportation phone numbers available should you need them. Make sure you have help to take care of other children or family pets so they don't get in the way. You need to concentrate on your labor, not what's going on around you. Your midwife or doula should give you instructions before the big day so you'll feel confident that your birth will be as natural as it can be without complications.

Spiritual Checklist for Hospital and Home Delivery

- Crystals
- Candles
- Essential oils
- Focal point item
- Your music playlist

- Herbal teas
- Flowers (buy these at the hospital or have someone bring your favorites ASAP)
- A throw for the hospital bed to mask the sterility
- Above all, a positive mind for a positive outcome

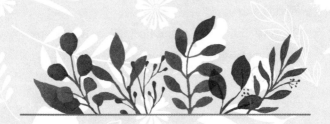

Weeks 38, 39, and 40

The perfect birth at the perfect time.

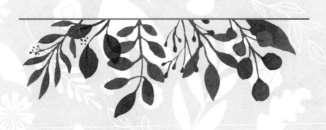

Baby—From now until the end of your pregnancy, there is not much going on with the baby except weight gain and gaining core strength. The brain is still developing and will continue to develop after birth. Womb space is at full capacity. The baby's movements are slower and more defined, unlike previous weeks where the baby had ample room to move. They now curl into an even tighter fetal position to accommodate any discomfort should it arise.

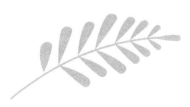

Mother—Everything is pretty much perfect. The clock is ticking, and you can't help but wonder when the birth will finally take place. Even if you've been given a due date, only five percent of babies are born on the scheduled date. Babies come when they are good and ready and not before unless there's a medical reason that needs an induced labor.

The bad thing about the wait is your discomfort. Your breasts feel heavy, your ankles swell, your back hurts, and you can't wear some of your rings or bracelets anymore. You may feel a little nauseous and tired and you might wonder if your toes are still there since you haven't seen them for a while.

You could also suffer from mood swings and may feel more vulnerable every day. Hug your partner or anyone that offers. Don't be shy and, if you feel like it, cry until your heart's content. Your hormones and mood swings dance inside you like a bad episode of *Dancing with the Stars*.

Flowers—White

In these final weeks, concentrate on white flowers. Their spiritual essence welcomes new life. They announce rebirth while you wait for the big reveal, which will be one of the most beautiful, rewarding, and emotional experiences of your life. This little bundle you carry wants to meet you just as much as you want to meet him or her.

Crystal—Rose Quartz

In week 30 we used rose quartz to spread love to the friends and loved ones you may have neglected due to work, tiredness, or wanting time with your baby and partner. This crystal is about unconditional love and mending bridges, not only with those we unconsciously abandoned or haven't seen for a while, but the abandonment we may feel within ourselves.

Rose quartz helps us understand the process of life and will ready you for the next chapter of your pregnancy and birth. Rose quartz brings a sense of peace and mystical wonder that will ease discomfort and complications should they manifest, while giving unconditional love to the birthing process and to your child.

You can add other crystals to the fray to help, such as aventurine for aches and pains, amethyst for discomfort, or another crystal you've learned to trust throughout the process of nurturing life.

Color—Soft Pastels

From now until labor, make soft pastels your color of choice. Pastels are gentle, soothing, and they bring comfort when needed. Pastels handle stressful situations with an ease that cools before emotions have time to fester or ignite. Think of light blues for comfort; pink for understanding; light yellow to strengthen your mind, body, and spirit; and white for faith in a loving delivery.

Chakra—Root

This chakra has carried you throughout your pregnancy and is now at its maximum frequency. At this point you could feel anxious, worried, excited, or tense, and you may feel physical discomfort. All of these could trigger a total disconnect from the other six chakras. This is normal and part of the birthing process. Until you go into labor, you'll find it difficult to stay grounded. How could you not? Excitement and wanting to meet the child you've lovingly carried for close to nine months is more than any sensory outlet can take. It can cause a little havoc with your state of mind and emotions.

Not knowing the outcome of a crucial situation in your life, like having a baby, causes fear within the root chakra. This can make you feel ungrounded and a tad spacey. This is totally normal, but you need to ground yourself. The more grounded you are, the better the emotional outcome throughout the delivery process will be.

Below are a few affirmations you can use throughout the next few weeks to bring your mind, body, and spirit back to equilibrium whenever you feel unsettled, worried, or simply want someone to tell you, "It's time to have this baby."

I am connected, I am grounded,
and I rejoice in the process of life's rituals.
I feel safe, secure, and excited to finally meet my child.
I feel confident in my ability
to go through the birthing process.
I rejoice in having a healthy birth.
I am wealthy with love and share its wealth
with those I love and the life that is soon to come forth.

Essential Oil—Mild

During these last few weeks, your nose may be able to tolerate essential oils better than before. Or it may only be able to handle a select few, or perhaps none at all. So, for these next few weeks, stick to the mild ones or one that stirs your senses and makes your home feel peaceful, while settling your mind so you can connect with your overjoyed spirit.

Use lavender to calm your internal countdown, frankincense to find spiritual awareness to connect with your inner goddess, and bergamot to lift your spirits. You can go back through previous weeks to find an essential oil that helped tame your heart and brought joy to a particular moment during your pregnancy.

Showers/Swimming

It may be a hassle to get in and out of the tub, even with someone's help. Stick to showers for the rest of your pregnancy. Take at least two a day to cool your body from the uncomfortable internal heat pregnancy seems to manifest, which can make you feel sticky and a little dusty and earthy. Use nice-scented bath gels and scrubs. Let the water heat your back to soften all those tight muscles and weary bones.

You can also go swimming. Swimming or floating takes away the weight of your body. It is also a great, gentle resistance exercise to strengthen your core muscles for the delivery. Swimming increases circulation and takes away back strain and sore muscles. And don't forget the buoyancy it gives you and the freedom it gives your body—making you feel like a large fluffy cloud.

Candles

Throughout the weeks you've used candles for all sorts of things, from seeking peace, courage, or forgiveness to finding love and understanding. They've even helped reassure the baby throughout their growth and development.

For these next three weeks or so, concentrate on courage, determination, and inner strength for you and the baby. Even if you're the one going through labor, the little life inside you is also working hard to meet you and finally leave its confined space.

Colored candles have a special meaning and find peace and courage within you. In these last few weeks, light red candles for courage, blue for peace, white for spiritual awareness, pink for love and understanding, green for healing and new experiences, and orange and yellow for intuition and creativity. When you see the flame of each candle, visualize the need you seek.

Meditation and Spiritual Boost

For the next few weeks, combine meditation with spiritual boosts. Visit family and friends and let them look after you. If your mother, mother-in-law, aunts, cousins, or friends want to cook for you and your partner or clean the house, let them. People need to feel useful in situations like these and you need to be pampered.

Go out for walks with your partner or friends. Get those legs moving to strengthen your muscles and help with your breathing. Look at nature and take in the best that life has to offer. Visualize walking with your baby safely snuggled in their stroller, breathing in all those past walks when they were in your tummy.

Keep doing your meditations. You can do them daily or weekly to find peace and comfort within you and your child. Meditation will clear the mind and keep you focused on your intention. Have your flowers in the background, light your candles, and allow the scent of your essential oil to awaken your senses. Play relaxing music that fills your soul. Go to your meditation space, turn down the lights, and find a comfortable position in your favorite chair or couch. Visualize the baby in their confined space. Talk to your child, venture to your womb, and embrace that little baby you have come to love so dearly. Gently touch their cheek and reassure them that life is wonderful and that you'll always be there for them.

From now on, you can also do quick meditations on the delivery. Visualize your doctor or midwife giving you precise instructions. Then, visualize yourself absorbing them like a sponge as you let them flow through your body with minimum pain and surprising ease.

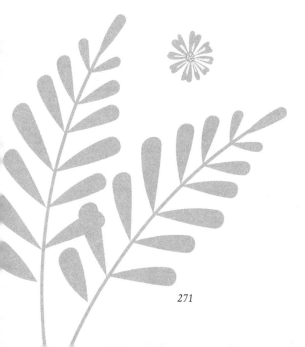

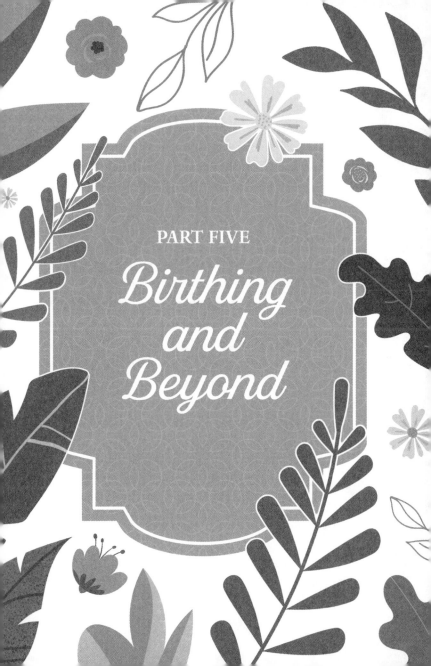

PART FIVE

Birthing and Beyond

The Birth

The pregnancy romance you've enjoyed during the past forty weeks will be the last chapter written in your journal after the birth of your baby. During the past nine months, you and your baby have readied for this moment. It's time to embrace the birth and meet the little bundle you've so gently nurtured.

You probably already know what to expect from your prenatal and birthing classes, but there is never enough planning that fully prepares you for birth. It's because we all experience the birthing process differently, even if this isn't your first child. You alone will know the emotions and discomforts you'll experience, but until that time, don't let the process of giving birth distract you from the experience. It's a rite of passage for billions of women worldwide. And guess what? You'll now join their ranks.

If you are giving birth in a hospital environment, it could feel a little sterile. After you've settled in with the baby monitor, gone through the hospital information about contractions, and found out about your dilation status, feel free to move around. Get as comfortable as you can and make the sterile hospital environment your own.

Find your Zen, just like you've been doing for the past forty weeks at home. Breathe as you've done during your meditations and concentrate on your root chakra, which at the present time is in chaos, unbalanced, scared, and could even make you feel unsafe. It's normal for the root chakra to act erratically as it prepares your emotions for the process of birth.

Getting the root chakra back to its functioning state is not as hard as you think. You need to coax it back to reality by reaffirming your intent, just like you've been doing since you found out you were pregnant.

Here are a few mantras for you to choose from. Pick one or several that apply to you.

- I am confident and I can handle the unknown with ease and comfort.
- I am grounded and feel the earth pulling me back to reality.
- Birth is powerful and it empowers me.
- I let my body guide me through this experience.
- I am worthy of a spiritual and loving labor.
- I can do this, and I am doing this.
- I listen to my birth team and feel safe in their care.
- This will not last forever.

Once you've selected your mantra(s), light the colored candle you've chosen for the birth and hold your preferred crystal. Place the throw over your hospital bed and let the aroma of your essential oil(s) comfort you and give you a sense of well-being, making you feel safe and comfortable. For the final touch, let someone go get you your favorite flowers. If you have no preference, let them get you white flowers to bring order, comfort, and peace into the delivery room. Even if disorder stirs with medical staff and your partner/birthing buddy, you can remain surprisingly calm. Focus completely on your body and your focal point, which needs to be within your sight line.

No one knows how long labor lasts. Some women take three hours while others take much longer, but once your medical team tells you to push one last time, a surge of energy within you flourishes the strength needed for that final act. I believe Mother Nature has given all women the strength for that final blessed push, which brings the baby out from confinement and into your arms.

The Placenta

The placenta is one of the most advanced organic filtering systems that has ever existed, but after the birth, this filtering and nurturing system is disposed of as medical waste in most hospitals unless you donate it to science.

We are developing ways to use the full potential of this magical organ's lining for burn victims and difficult-to-heal wounds such as diabetic ulcers. These afflictions benefit greatly from the amniotic membrane, as it heals and acts as an anti-inflammatory agent. The amniotic membrane is also used to help the healing process for various types of surgical procedures. Even the umbilical cord has critical uses for cancer patients.

There is no denying the unmistakable power the placenta offered while providing everything your baby needed while developing in your womb. While you hold your baby in your arms—healthy, beautiful, and safe—it makes you realize how wonderful the miracle of life can be.

If you have decided to keep the placenta as an offering to nature, you are not the only one in a growing spiritual society. There are cultures around the world that believe the placenta is sacred and should be given back to nature in a burial ritual. Some new mothers lay it flat on a large white piece of paper to imprint its tree-of-life appearance. They keep it as a symbol of respect for the journey it has taken, which will never be forgotten.

It's up to you how you wish to dispose of your placenta. If you want to dispose of it yourself, just remember you can't put it in a plastic bag and walk out of the hospital. If only it was that easy. Arrangements must be made beforehand because the placenta is a decaying organ and needs to be refrigerated until its disposal. Other things need to be considered, like wearing surgical gloves while handling it. Make sure to wash and disinfect your hands if you accidentally touch the placenta without gloves. In some countries you need a permit for its burial, which stipulates location and the depth it's to be buried.

If you've decided to bury it, prepare a small ritual. Thank it for your healthy baby and give it back to nature for the circle of life to begin again. After you've dug the hole and placed it gently into the earth, add a bunch of poinsettias, bluebells, or pink roses. All these flowers express gratitude and respect.

If you are interested in donating your placenta, contact an organ or tissue-donating agency in your part of the world.

Breastfeeding

One of the questions you'll be asked at the hospital is if you're going to breastfeed your baby. If you are, the nursing staff will not attempt to bottle-feed your baby so the baby only uses your nipple. If you are not going to breastfeed due to medical and prescription medication reasons, there are infant formulas with all the nutrients and vitamins the baby needs for their growth and development. You'll also get to experience the wonderful bonding cuddles close to your breasts while bottle-feeding.

The breastfeeding experience starts the moment you put your baby to your breast. When the baby finally latches, everything falls into place, but don't get discouraged if it takes a few times to get it right. At first, the process of breastfeeding can be frustrating, not only for you but for the baby as well. Get help from the breastfeeding nurse at the hospital. If you're at home, your midwife or doula can guide you through techniques that are best for both of you.

Breast milk is not only nutritionally good for your baby but is also helps you lose weight and activates the hormones that help the uterus contract back to its normal size. Breastfeeding can be a natural contraceptive as well as being economically sound with a new baby in the home.

You can use crystals like moonstone and rose quartz to help with the bonding experience while breastfeeding. For breast milk to flow in abundance, carry crystals such as white calcite, fluorite, and apatite. They will help you relax and allow you to let Mother Nature take over the oldest means of nurturing and bonding with your child.

Mothering the Mother After Birth

If you're a first-time mother, the experience is not only challenging, but foreign. You've just had this gorgeous little baby who has you awake most of the night crying, wanting to be fed, and to be kept dry or be cuddled. You're exhausted and emotionally drained. You may start to feel your life is out of control and you might second-guess yourself about everything. If breastfeeding is still difficult, it can take its toll and make you wonder what happened to the peace and enlightenment you felt over the past forty weeks.

The way you feel is absolutely normal. Your body is coming down from one of the biggest hormonal highs a woman will ever go through. You've just had a baby. You're probably still tired from the birth, not to mention teary if you had a difficult labor. And if you had a caesarean birth, you're sore and uncomfortable.

Your body is physically, mentally, and emotionally trying to get back to where it was before the baby was born. You also want to bond with your child, but you might second-guess yourself, which can turn your doubts into fear. You might ask yourself repeatedly, "Am I doing the right thing for the baby?" This question unconsciously becomes a battle cry deep within you and needs to be heard.

You probably want the world to see that you're happy and adore your sweet little baby when in truth you're in need of cuddles and reassurance yourself. But you're too busy comforting your crying baby who might not stop no matter what you do. It may make you think you're doing it all wrong. This is what's referred to as the baby blues, which is a natural part of the birth aftermath. So please don't make people think you're coping if you're not.

The first thing to do is tell someone how overwhelmed you feel. The first person to tell is the person who has taken the journey of creating life with you. Talk to your partner, who is trying to adjust to parenting just as much as you are, and tell them how you feel. Find a way to work together to help each other. Share responsibility. If you are breastfeeding, let your partner change the baby and then bring the baby to you. If you are not breastfeeding, share the bottle-feeding. You can always find a way to work together by communicating your needs and sharing the workload and responsibilities as a unit rather than individuals.

You can always call in the big guns: the women on both sides of the family. Your mother and partner's mother expect to be called in to help. If they don't live close, ask friends or a trusted neighbor. You'll be surprised at how many people want to help. Let them know their help is needed and wanted. Don't be shy and ask for help. People will answer your plea with open arms.

Let those that want to help clean your house, cook, and even go to the market or run errands. Let them do the endless loads of laundry and take care of the baby while you sneak in a nap after breastfeeding. The extra rest will do wonders for your emotions, your body, and your state of mind. Once you reach that state of mind, you begin to trust yourself and your motherly instincts surface to take control of the journey, making it more rewarding and less stressful.

It's important after you bring your baby home to keep in touch with your medical provider. If you are not coping even while getting help and support, please seek medical advice. You could be suffering from postpartum depression, which is common and treated successfully; you just need to ask for help to find your way back to your loved ones and that gorgeous new baby you love so much.

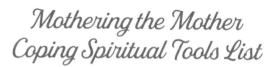

Mothering the Mother
Coping Spiritual Tools List

Candles: White, purple, and pink
Essential Oils: Lavender, lemon, and bergamot
Flowers: Any pink flowers for love, peace,
and bonding
Crystals: Amethyst, rose quartz, moonstone,
or aventurine
Colors: Purple, blue, white, or pink
Chakra: Root chakra affirmation:

> *I am strong and I am a good mother.*
> *No one is judging me.*

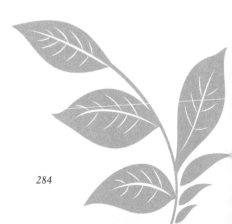

Baby Past-Life Memories

It's important to keep past lives in mind after your baby is born. Your baby is still oblivious of anything to do with past lives, but your baby's soul isn't. Your baby's soul has just taken total possession and is ready to learn and correct previous past lives in this life. The amnesia has not taken effect, and everything is vivid as though it happened yesterday. Eventually, these memories will fade as your child grows. The chances of them remembering any past-life experiences in their future are slim unless they go into hypnotic therapy.

Until that time comes, it's helpful to know the little soul you hold dear may have gone through a traumatic event in a past life. The baby doesn't understand these emotions or why they're invading its space. They react by not settling down or waking up in a screaming frenzy. It's because the baby doesn't understand the process of life yet. How could they? It's like trying to teach a toddler math.

When your baby doesn't settle down and isn't hungry, wet, or tired, your maternal instincts kick in and you'll ask yourself, "Is the baby sick or seeking comfort?" When this happens, hold your baby and know they could have an uncomfortable past-life memory and because they can't voice how they feel, they'll cry or whimper. You can comfort them by holding them tightly.

Make your baby feel they are loved. Put a rose quartz inside a sock and hide it somewhere in the crib to settle the baby and to help them find comfort. You can hang a dream catcher by their crib to catch the bad dreams or memories. When you soothe your baby, rock them back to sleep while saying:

Everything is as it should be, calm and at peace.
You are in loving arms
and forever will be.

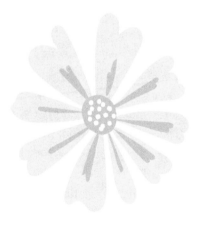

Monday's Child

The Spiritual Birth Week

Depending on which day of the week your child is born on, the following may attribute to your child's character.

Monday's child: Intuitive and bright

Tuesday's child: Courageous and wise

Wednesday's child: Problem-solver and judge

Thursday's child: Lawyer and legal diplomat

Friday's child: Friend and lover for life

Saturday's child: Seeker of truth and justice

Sunday's child: Healer of physical and spiritual life

Baby Birthstones

January: Garnet

February: Amethyst

March: Aquamarine

April: Diamond

May: Emerald

June: Pearl

July: Ruby

August: Peridot

September: Sapphire

October: Opal, Tourmaline

November: Topaz, Citrine

December: Zircon, Turquoise

Your Child's Star Signs

Aries: March 21 to April 19
Crystal: Blood Stone
Fire Sign
THE RAM

Aries children are fun, active in sports, and driven by anything that catches their attention until the next thing comes along for them to explore. They charm anyone with their charismatic personality and their leadership abilities on the playground. They are smart and quick learners if it's something they're interested in. They like the attention of their mothers, they share toys easily, and freely express their emotions.

Taurus: April 20 to May 20
Crystal: Sapphire
Earth Sign
THE BULL

Tauruses are loyal and dependable children. They can be cautious and indulge in things they like. They can be volcanic, but cool off as quickly as they ignite. The Taurus child can be hard to reason with at times, but with coaxing they'll come around ... eventually. They are very grounded and are not followers, but leaders.

They love music, so make sure it's a part of their world. They love attention and crave cuddles and playtime with mom and dad.

Gemini: May 21 to June 21
Crystal: Agate
Air Sign
THE TWINS

Little Geminies get distracted easily and abandon one game for another at a second's notice, but when they stick to something, there's no stopping them. They are very smart, resourceful, and little social butterflies. They excel in sports they enjoy. They are chatterboxes, and they constantly ask questions to satisfy their curiosity. They are creative and will swoop you into their fantasy play. When encouraged, there is nothing your Gemini can't do.

Cancer: June 22 to July 22
Crystal: Emerald
Water Sign
THE CRAB

Cancer babies are full of love and are very affectionate and friendly. They're very social and crave parental love. They will stand up for those that are bullied and act bravely in the process. They are little jokesters and remember everything. They can be sensitive, and this makes you want to protect them and give them the emotional stability they need. When you do, the reward you'll receive is heartwarming.

Leo: July 23 to August 22
Crystal: Onyx
Fire Sign
THE LION

Children born under the sign of Leo are great conversationalists and always cheerful. They have natural leadership qualities and they are competitive in everything they do. Little Leos love competitive sports, which help to wear them out. They are affectionate and love animals—any animal. They give out lots of hugs and kisses and expect them back. Nurture them and you'll be surprised at what's under that academically or artistically talented personality.

Virgo: August 23 to September 22
Crystal: Carnelian
Earth Sign
THE VIRGIN

Virgos are the healers of the star signs—smart and challenging. They need plenty of rest due to their active personalities and intellectual demands. They are very grounded and benefit from order and schedules. Little Virgos are responsible, and they want to make you proud of them, so praise them when praise is due. This makes them feel good about themselves and they'll keep excelling so you'll continue to be proud of them.

Libra: September 23 to October 22
Crystal: Peridot
Air Sign
THE SCALES

A Libra child is creative in everything they do. They are intelligent, especially when they feel balanced. They see both sides of the story and never judge. It may take a Libra child time to get dressed because they can't pick an outfit. They like company and like to please. They lose track of time when they're engaged in activities they love. Being an air sign, they are very creative and love music from all genres and ages. Nurture their artistic flare, which will flourish in later years.

Scorpio: October 23 to November 21
Crystal: Aquamarine
Water Sign
THE SCORPION

Little Scorpios are dreamers and can be competitive at times, as well as creative. They like to study things that interest them and excel when they do. They love and care deeply. They can be a little possessive at times, which can be challenging, but patience and reassurance is all they need. Be honest with your Scorpio child and know they can be a little mysterious and emotionally intense at times, but very loving and loyal to a fault.

Sagittarius: November 22 to December 21
Crystal: Topaz
Fire Sign
THE ARCHER

You will need to watch your little Sagittarius—they are constantly on the move. They make sure to tell you what they want. They don't identify with fear, so don't turn your back on them because they'll cause mischief. They like car trips because they give them time to explore their surroundings and nature. They are funny and defiant, so be prepared for the challenges while you nurture their insistent, loving little Saggi personality.

Capricorn—December 22 to January 19
Crystal: Ruby
Earth Sign
THE GOAT

Little Capricorns are great thinkers. They are very responsible and seem older than they are at times. They are absorbers and analyzers. They can be a little shy, but once they get to know you, love shines within them and there's no stopping the openness to their personality. They are hard workers, diligent, loyal, and enjoy tasks, which they complete to the best of their capabilities.

Aquarius—January 20 to February 18
Crystal: Garnet
Air Sign
THE WATER BEARER

Aquarians are a social and outgoing bunch. They are great thinkers and very loyal to their friends. They will ask you the same question over and over again until they get an answer, so be ready for them. This star sign is busy and on-the-go. Things need to make sense to an Aquarian, and if something doesn't, they get frustrated. Letting them vent is the key to your own emotional peace.

Pisces—February 19 to March 20
Crystal: Amethyst
Water Sign
THE FISH

Pisceans are dreamers. They don't like to get dirty and get stuck in la-la land quite often. They are great at make-believe playtime because they're more creative than physical. They like to feel connected to the family collective, where they'll excel with love and support. It's so important for your little Piscean to be heard, so make sure to listen and follow up with lots of cuddles.

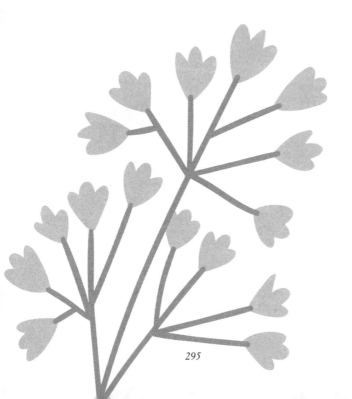

Closing

As parents, we have the power to shape the future of mankind, so be kind, treat your child with respect, and give them a voice. Be there for all the happy and stressful and emotional moments in your child's life. Your child has had the most wondrous, healthy, and loving womb experience. Be assured the baby you now hold will have a life full of possibilities and encouraging outcomes.

Family Mantra

A decision made together as a family
is always the right decision.

~Ileana

Further Reading and Information

Books

The Day-by-Day Pregnancy Book

Dr. Maggie Blott and Professor Jonathan Morris,
updated edition published in Australia 2018 by
DK—Penguin / Random House

What to Expect When You Are Expecting

Heidi Muroff, first Australian publication 1987, by
Angus and Robertson Publishers and Harper
Collins

Guide to a Healthy Pregnancy

Mayo Clinic, published 2011 by The Pregnancy Experts
at Mayo Clinic

Online

https://www.parents.com

https://techigem.com/period-tracker-apps

https://www.pregnancybirthbaby.org.au/what-to-
take-to-hospital-checklist

https://www.huggies.com

Further Listening

Spotify Playlists

Baby Sleep: Soothing instrumental music for sleepy
babies.
This is a mixture of all genres with a classical feel to it.

*Babies' Bedtime:*100% Natural Sleep Aid & Nursery
Melodies.
This is a mixture of older popular songs, both calming
and soothing.

To Write to the Author

If you wish to contact the author or would like more information about this book, please write to the author in care of Llewellyn Worldwide Ltd. and we will forward your request. Both the author and publisher appreciate hearing from you and learning of your enjoyment of this book and how it has helped you. Llewellyn Worldwide Ltd. cannot guarantee that every letter written to the author can be answered, but all will be forwarded. Please write to:

Ileana Abrev
℅ Llewellyn Worldwide
2143 Wooddale Drive
Woodbury, MN 55125-2989

Please enclose a self-addressed stamped envelope for reply, or $1.00 to cover costs. If outside the U.S.A., enclose an international postal reply coupon.

Many of Llewellyn's authors have websites with additional information and resources.

For more information, please visit our website at http://www.llewellyn.com